PRAISE FOR

Fit, Fun and Fabulous
At Any Age

AND DR. KATHLEEN HARTFORD

Dr. Kathleen Hartford has a unique ability to bridge the understanding between traditional and natural healthcare. She accomplishes this through a scientifically based integrated approach that moves her clients toward wellness care. Her positive and engaging approach is refreshing in the age of misinformation and confusion in health and wellness choices.

—Freddie H. Fu, MD
Chairman, Department of Orthopaedic Surgery,
University of Pittsburgh Medical Center

Dr. Kathleen Hartford is a chiropractor by education and training but so much more. She integrates chiropractic techniques with Eastern philosophy and Western medicine. A beautiful person both inside and outside, Dr. Kathy encourages everyone to be the best they can be, and she emanates positive energy to everyone who comes in contact with her.

—Ruby Kang
Health and Wellness Coordinator,
Ladies Hospital Aid Society

Fit, Fun and Fabulous *is a remarkable program for anyone who doesn't know where to begin their journey into weight loss and healthy living. The program is clear and concise. It will truly help you recognize and understand the benefits of a healthy lifestyle. Kudos to Dr. Hartford!*

—Lindsey Smith
Holistic Health Coach,
Author and Owner of *The Real You*

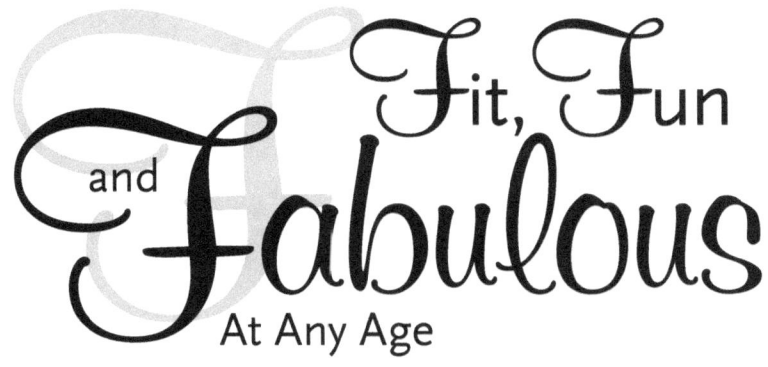

Fit, Fun and Fabulous
At Any Age

A 12-Week
Rejuvenation Program
for the Rest of Your Life

DR. KATHLEEN A. HARTFORD

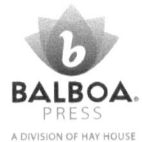

BALBOA.
PRESS

A DIVISION OF HAY HOUSE

Balboa Press books may be ordered through booksellers or by contacting:

Balboa Press
A Division of Hay House
1663 Liberty Drive
Bloomington, IN 47403
www.balboapress.com
1-(877) 407-4847

Because of the dynamic nature of the Internet, any web addresses or links contained in this book may have changed since publication and may no longer be valid. The views expressed in this work are solely those of the author and do not necessarily reflect the views of the publisher, and the publisher hereby disclaims any responsibility for them.

The author of this book does not dispense medical advice or prescribe the use of any technique as a form of treatment for physical, emotional, or medical problems without the advice of a physician, either directly or indirectly. The intent of the author is only to offer information of a general nature to help you in your quest for emotional and spiritual well-being. In the event you use any of the information in this book for yourself, which is your constitutional right, the author and the publisher assume no responsibility for your actions.

Certain stock imagery © Thinkstock.
Any people depicted in stock imagery provided by Thinkstock are models, and such images are being used for illustrative purposes only.

ISBN: 978-1-4525-3387-2 (e)
ISBN: 978-1-4525-3386-5 (sc)
ISBN: 978-1-4525-3388-9 (hc)

Library of Congress Control Number: 2011906315

Printed in the United States of America

Balboa Press rev. date: 5/18/2011

Cover Art – Martha Wasik
Editors – Gina Mazza and Linda Martin

To Khalehla, my daughter and my "smile."
You are perfect and beautiful in every way.

To my husband, Dr. William F. Donaldson III,
for your continuous love and support and your amazing ability
to make me laugh every day.

To my grandmother, Concetta, who implored me at age 19
to help my parents understand the importance of nutrition.
Grandma, this book is a testament to my love for you—and don't worry,
Mom and Dad are just fine.

To my parents and my brothers for loving me unconditionally.
Perhaps my most endearing moment was when my father acknowledged
that all of the non-conventional things concerning health that he has
heard me say over the years, he's now heard about on the evening
news ... or better yet, read about in the *Wall Street Journal.*

ACKNOWLEDGEMENTS

I would like to take this opportunity to acknowledge my professional mentors, who have always worked outside the box to create new realms of possibilities in the healthcare arena:

Dr. Verne Pierce, my father in structural chiropractic, for the most effective analysis through motion picture X-ray and the most freeing adjusting technique for the spine, dura and nervous system that I have yet to find. "Correct the subluxations and the compensations will take care of themselves!"

Dr. Victor Frank, my father in healing, who continuously proved that "the Power that made the body can heal the body." Create balance and all else will follow. He took healing out of cadaver physiology into functional physiology to create miracles for all he touched and all he taught.

Dr. Scott Walker, who had the vision to create Neuro-Emotional Technique. NET works with laser focus on the origins of so many of our mind patterns and limited belief structures that create pain, suffering and paralysis in our lives. It is a must for anyone wanting to integrate body, mind and spirit in a compassionate and enlightened way.

Dr. Guy Riekeman, President of Life University is perhaps the most eloquent orator of vitalism in the world today. Dr. Riekeman has lived his life 'on purpose' while maintaining the integrity of Chiropractic as a Philosophy, Science and an Art. "While the philosophy is always an ideal and the living is always flawed, it is in the striving toward the ideal that creates vision, power and inspiration." As humans we are flawed but it is in striving toward the ideal that we can create our best lives while reaching and maintaining our optimum genetic expression of health. Keep Dr. Riekeman's words in mind as you begin your journey toward wellness.

Dr. Jeffrey Bland, whose work I admire and utilize in my practice, as well as in my *Fit, Fun and Fabulous* program; he is a renowned biochemist and leader in the fields of functional medicine, nutritional medicine and systems biology. He continues to take functional nutrition to levels never before seen—creating healing systems that, if incorporated, will alter the course of healthcare. I deeply believe that failing to incorporate his techniques and protocols into medicine is negligence.

Special thanks to all of my patients, most of whom have been with me for years. I appreciate your continued commitment and dedication to maintaining the highest level of health possible for yourselves and your families.

To my staff and, in particular, Melody—for all you do and especially for our companion *Fit, Fun and Fabulous Cookbook.*

Finally, special thanks to Gina Mazza, Linda Martin, Holly Wensel at NPS, and Martha Wasik for creating the beautiful words, images and designs that comprise this book.

CONTENTS

INTRODUCTION

Congratulations! You have made a commitment to experiencing this Biological Rejuvenation Program, and this means that you now hold in your hands the key to remaining *Fit, Fun and Fabulous* at any age. My personal promise to you is that by the time you complete the steps outlined in this book, you will be well on your way to enjoying a more vibrant and healthy life. You will feel better, look younger, be more relaxed and have increased energy to do all the things that are important to you in life.

We'll cover exciting and important subject matter in this lifestyle program, with an emphasis on what makes you sick, what makes your body age and how you can, in fact, decelerate that aging process. How is this possible? The steps for doing so are based around *12 Biomarkers of Aging* that have been identified by scientists at Tufts University. The very exciting news is that all 12 of these indicators can be positively influenced by three basic areas that are in your control: nutrition, exercise and quality rest.

Briefly, the 12 biomarkers are:

1. Body cell mass (the lean muscle composition of your body)
2. Strength (your musculoskeletal fitness)
3. Basal metabolic rate
4. Body fat composition
5. Body fat distribution
6. Aerobic capacity

7. Blood sugar tolerance

8. Level of cholesterol / HDL ratio

9. Blood pressure

10. Internal temperature regulation

11. Bone mineral density

12. Resting heart rate

This Biological Rejuvenation Program includes an in-depth look at each of the biomarkers and how working with them can halt or reverse the accelerated aging process. I invite you to review the individual biomarkers in the appendix of this book. There is a bit more technical information there, some of which is covered in the body of this text and some that is not. My purpose is to outline a health-enhancing lifestyle to stop the accelerated aging process, which occurs as these biomarkers shift. If you're interested in losing weight, following this program will absolutely achieve that for you but this program will also reframe things for you. You will discover that, instead of losing weight in order to become healthy, *the weight loss occurs naturally after good health is achieved.* Healthy people do not maintain excessive fat deposits in their bodies—only unhealthy bodies created by unhealthy lifestyle choices do.

Here is a quick rundown of the lifestyle topics that comprise this Biological Rejuvenation Program:

- Biological versus chronological age, and the importance of having a biological age assessment
- Healthy eating habits and the importance of eating frequently to stabilize blood sugar
- Syndrome X (better known as metabolic syndrome or insulin resistance) and determining if you or your children might have this and therefore be at risk of becoming a type 2 diabetic
- The body in motion and the biomechanical realities of bone and joint health
- The importance of exercise and which types of exercises are vital to reverse the biomarkers of aging
- Good stress versus bad stress and the emotional, biochemical and energetic effects of both types of stress

- Relaxation and the need for downtime, along with various types of relaxation techniques
- Hormone balancing for both women and men
- Body shapes, including where you hold your weight and what this fat distribution means in terms of stress on the organs and body systems
- Targeted supplementation with vitamins and nutrients—how to determine what is good, what is necessary, which nutrients should be taken together or apart, and why some should be taken with food and others on an empty stomach, as they relate to this program

Finally, we will finish the program with a summary of your biological age assessment to show that you can be biologically younger this year than last. We want to be able to chart your progress, and the biological age indicators will help us do just that.

So, get ready! It's going to be a revolutionary time. If you follow these lifestyle changes, you can become biologically younger within just weeks, but you shouldn't stop there. You can maintain your biological youth and vitality for a lifetime. Enjoy the journey to better health and a more vibrant you!

Chapter 1

NEW BEGINNINGS

The Biological Rejuvenation Program that you are about to undertake will change the biological aspect of your body called "functional physiology." My experience with patients has shown me that changing your biology can create a shift in your entire life—physically, spiritually and emotionally.

You are not a compartmentalized machine; you are a whole being whose parts are interrelated and adapting to each other every second of every day. When you think a thought, you change your body's chemistry via neuropeptides, which give information to your cells, tissues and organs. We have all experienced a difference in our physical bodies when the information we tell ourselves is "I feel happy, fit and accomplished" versus "I feel sad, sluggish and undervalued." Everything you say, eat, do or are is received as information in your body. Your body responds to the information it is given, and that data comes in the forms of: the food you eat, the thoughts you think, the water you drink, the exercise you choose to participate in, and more. Knowing this is dynamic and exciting, because it puts the power of your life experiences—physically, spiritually and emotionally—directly in your hands!

Given the fact that our human bodies operate in a holistic manner, I recommend that everyone consider a whole-body approach to their health and wellness routines, which often times falls outside the realm of traditional medicine. By its very nature, traditional medicine must be practiced in a compartmentalized way due to the depth of knowledge required to treat a disease or address a surgical condition. Case in point: you would not want your surgeon to assume the duties of your primary care physician, pharmacist, internist and anesthesiologist on the day of surgery. You would want each of these physicians available to focus on his/her own area of specialization, and to do it extremely well. If they lost focus, you could die.

Unfortunately, when it comes to maintaining health and wellness, I'm afraid this compartmentalized approach does not work. Chronic disease rates are sharply rising and the latest published study from Health Affairs revealed that the United States now ranks 49th for male and female life expectancy worldwide. This is down dramatically from 5th place in the 1950s. The chronic diseases that are killing us include diabetes, heart disease, obesity and cancer. They are rampant in our country and in many parts of our world. The purpose of this book is to educate you on the factors that cause and contribute to these chronic diseases and to return the power of health to your hands.

True health care is integrated wellness care that must be utilized in the hands of those best trained to do so. Traditional medicine is effective when dealing with emergency treatment, but I believe that the arena of total healthcare would be greatly enriched by merging traditional methods with those of the holistic practitioner. My vision for the future is traditional and natural healthcare practitioners working hand in hand to support their patients' whole health needs by focusing on and acknowledging each other's respective areas of competency. Throughout this book I will stress the differences between the traditional primary care provider and a natural healthcare provider. A natural or holistic physician sees your body as more than the sum of your parts and specializes in balancing those parts, to maintain normal healthy function. Natural health practitioners are interested in the *prevention* and *reversal* of dis-ease, whether for health maintenance, reversing a dis-ease process, preparing you for a necessary surgery or supporting your healing process post-surgically. The dash in "dis-ease" is an important distinction between these two types of health practitioners. Integrative natural health practitioners identify where the body has lost its ease of healthy function and entered a state of "lack of ease of function" or "dis-ease." Medical doctors are trained to detect the disease state where the body no longer is *able* to perform appropriate function. Remember, the disease process occurs over time, beginning first with dis-ease. If we can distinguish it at the point of "dis-ease" then we can prevent disease! That is the approach we will take as we work together through this Biological Rejuvenation Program.

Before You Begin

Before starting your life enhancement journey, please be sure to do the following things:

Sign the Agreements

First, sign the *My Agreement* form (located at the end of this chapter). This is an agreement that you will make only with yourself. By doing this in writing, it will become more concrete, and you will be formally affirming to yourself that living with vibrant health is now your priority.

Next, complete the *My Life Assessment* form (also located at the end of this chapter). This will help bring into focus your feelings about your present life—where you feel successful and at ease, and where you feel challenged and unhappy. As you clean up your internal life, you will find that many of your external issues will become clearer as well. Remember that life is a balancing act, and any imbalance will eventually create internal disharmony. At the same time, if you change the dynamic of any part of a system (especially for the better), the whole system will change.

Keep a Journal

As you work through new topics in each section of this book, I strongly recommend that you use your personal journal to record your progress, as well as your thoughts and feelings. This journal will become your close friend and confidant over the course of the program. Please use it to its maximum potential as a way to reinforce your commitment to the program and, more importantly, to honor your vow to take better care of your body, mind and spirit from today forward. For your convenience, we offer a nifty purse-sized companion journal to this book that you can take with you everywhere. Order it at <drkathleenhartford.com>.

The Biological Rejuvenation Program is a lifestyle program. It is essential that the required changes are integrated into your daily life choices. Each day, you will be asked to use your journal to record all of the foods that you've eaten—the good, the bad and the ugly—from the *Anti-inflammatory Food Schedule* (in the Appendix). This list is vitally important to reverse the biomarkers of aging and to slow the aging process. In fact, most diseases begin as the result of increased inflammation in your system. You will no doubt hear during the coming years that all diseases—from cancer, to infection to heart disease—are connected to the inflammatory processes within the body. What causes inflammation? It can be caused by many things, but the one thing that we have direct and complete control over every day is the inflammatory food that we put into our bodies. That is why I am asking you to keep a record of everything you ingest until this knowledge becomes second nature to you.

As you work through the program each day, you will also be asked to complete the remaining questions in your journal and then "release" the day. What's done is done, so let it go. If you've had an especially bad day with the program or some other aspect of your life, determine the root cause and why it took you off course. Was it a relationship or work issue, another stress, a physical ailment or pain, PMS or a severe headache? Was there an opportunity within this perceived problem where you had the power of choice to change the dynamic? If so, what could you have chosen to do differently? Journal about that. Is there a time when your only source of power is to make peace with the way things are? If that is the case, journal about that as well.

If you get stuck while in the midst of this journaling process, please know that you can schedule a coaching session at <drkathleenhartford. com>. We all have challenging times in our lives, and utilizing a coach is an excellent way to get through difficult moments. I only ask that you be open to being powerful and exploring opportunities for change—whether it's a change of heart, a story that you've bought into or a change of mind. Coaching is about enabling you to form the habit of saying "yes" to yourself, and I will support your efforts to achieve that goal. Please remember, there is only one person in any equation that you can change, and that person is you. You must say "yes" to you! Our power is great when it is focused; the purpose of your journal is to help you achieve and maintain that focus.

Get Online Support

While following this program, feel free to visit <drkathleenhartford.com> at any time, and listen to podcasts covering topics from food to relationships. Behavior modification takes time and repetition, so do whatever works best for you to help integrate this information until it is second nature to you. Listening to podcasts, along with journaling and reading, all activate different areas of learning.

A Special Word to Parents

Moms and dads, please consider extending this program to your children by making it the lifestyle for your family. Feed them the same food that you eat, and they will reap the same rewards that you reap. As the caregivers of our children, we set an important example, and their health will be largely determined by the choices we make: the activities we participate in, the food we purchase, and the restaurants we frequent. You are the most influential person in their lives, so make a commitment to acknowledge that responsibility in a powerful new way, beginning right now.

To help you and your family make a seamless transition to becoming healthier, our certified organic chef, Melody Pierce, has created the companion *Fit, Fun and Fabulous Cookbook*. It contains a variety of delicious recipes that are packed with high quality nutrients. To get additional recipes and other healthy tidbits, you can sign up for our free weekly newsletter at <drkathleenhartford.com>.

I am excited about the opportunities that lie ahead for you and your family as you embark on this lifestyle program. Your best results will come when you follow the protocols, ask for help when needed, journal your experiences and exercise (begin to feel your body move and be grateful for that). You are truly blessed if you have the means to buy groceries, so why not use the guidelines outlined in this book to purchase the best quality food for yourself and your family? Now is the time to begin! Go forward with a positive attitude, gratitude and determination.

*Note: For a daily outline of meal suggestions to make your first week easier please visit www.fitfunandfabulous.com

A Typical Fit, Fun and Fabulous Day

Here is a preview of how your typical day will look from this day forward. Begin by doing the following:

- Go to your food list in the Appendix and shop for the appropriate health-supportive foods.
- Set your alarm clock 15 minutes earlier than normal.
- Explore the type of exercise that you would enjoy, or begin today with walking.
- Ask a friend or family member if they'd like to do this program with you.
- Review the use of your journal.
- Use your extra 15 -20 minutes to enjoy morning quiet time for reflection and journaling.

Okay, stop laughing! It is important to understand that our bodies need this quiet time. It gives our bodies the opportunity to consciously balance our sympathetic and parasympathetic nervous systems. When we begin our day being catapulted out of bed with our hearts and minds already racing, we release certain biochemicals. One such biochemical, for example, is cortisol, a steroid hormone produced by the adrenal gland in response to stress. Its primary functions are to increase blood sugar through gluconeogenesis (see Biomarkers 1 and 2), suppress the immune system, and aid in fat, protein and carbohydrate metabolism. It also decreases bone formation, which contributes to osteopenia and osteoporosis. Its presence over the long term has a negative effect on all of the biomarkers of aging and therefore needs to be managed.

You may be wondering, *How on earth do I control a steroid that my body creates?* Well, here comes the importance of self-induced quiet time. In clinical terms, it involves switching from the sympathetic nervous system (fight or flight) to the parasympathetic nervous system (healing, relaxation and repair), We all know that prolonged stress is detrimental to the body on every level, so if starting and ending our day with a period of quiet repose, shifts us from stress (cortisol-filled fight or flight) to peace (serotonin-filled healing, relaxation and repair), then the importance of it becomes clear. I will discuss this in more detail in a later chapter.

When you were completing the *My Life Assessment* form, I asked you to sit quietly and focus on your breathing. As you did that, you were to strive to become aware of your inner core and simply "be" with yourself. Some people do this as a meditation, some as a prayer, and some use this time to journal and set their sights for the day. I ask that you spend 15 to 20 minutes every morning doing this in whatever manner you choose. You will be amazed at the difference in your day. (In fact, please email me and share your experience. I'd love to hear about it.) If stress is something that you feel is out of control in your life, explore more opportunities at the Institute of HeartMath (Heartmath.org). Their techniques will greatly assist your morning quiet time and help to minimize your stress throughout the day.

Exercise

Exercise for a minimum of three days per week, 30 minutes each workout. If you have not been exercising, you may want to start with a brisk walk and slowly work your way into some form of weight-resistance exercises with light weights or bands. Pilates or yoga are also wonderful for flexibility and core strength. Please explore various forms of exercise at <drkathleenhartford.com> and if your financial position allows, consider fitness coaching, advice from a personal trainer, or join a gym or studio that has structured classes. (This is where I have to write a disclaimer stating that you should see your doctor before beginning an exercise program ... so please do so!)

As you master the three-day-a-week workouts, you may have a desire to do more (I would love to see five!), which would be even better. If possible, walk each day whenever you can fit it into your schedule. It may be convenient to walk at lunch during the workday or with a loved one after dinner. Some women find it to be a great way to spend time with their friends, and it really does beat sitting in a coffee shop. A walking meditation is an excellent way to start or end your day.

Journaling

Please commit to using your journal *every day*. I cannot stress enough the importance of using your own words as a promise to yourself. Journaling will help you to be clear on your commitment to create a *Fit, Fun and Fabulous* life, and it will help you to spot behaviors that might distract you from your goals. Please fill in every line of your journal. If this is difficult or if you see a repetitive pattern that continuously takes you away from this promise to yourself, please email me at <drkathleenhartford.com> for some personal coaching to work through those behavior patterns or to find a coach near you. If your behavior is self-destructive or hurts others, please find a therapist with whom you would be comfortable working. Through my chiropractic practice, I often see just how emotionally wounded we all may be, some of us more than others. If those wounds have you acting out in destructive ways, then please seek help.

Five Meals Per Day

Your five meals would be breakfast, lunch and dinner with a mid-morning and mid-afternoon snack. Choose food from your food guide, or select a meal replacement drink or protein bar that is micro- (vitamins and minerals) and macro- (proteins, carbohydrates and fat) nutrient balanced. These are available at <drkathleenhartford.com> but please use them for no more than two snack meals a day unless under a doctor's supervision. Use recipes from our companion *Fit, Fun and Fabulous Cookbook* or from the free newsletter that we mail each week (sign up at <drkathleenhartford. com>). There are other equally wonderful healthy cookbooks available, as well. I personally do not use cookbooks, as everything on my dinner plate is simply prepared. I get my starch from high quality rice, legumes and beans, add a huge portion of my favorite vegetables and a protein portion the size of the palm of my hand—simple, clean and easy. I drizzle a little olive oil, sea salt and herbs to taste, and I'm good to go. Give your taste buds a week of clean, healthy food, and you will never go back to those heavy foods and sauces.

Vitamins and Supplements

If you are currently taking vitamins and other supplements, check their labels for a GMP certification. This assures that what is on the label is actually in the bottle. There are many low-quality nutrients on the shelves of various stores. My suggestion would be to visit your local licensed natural healthcare practitioner (one that your family members or friends love), and speak to him/her about physician-only supplement lines. The targeted nature of these products will far outperform most products on the market. Avoid getting your nutritional guidance from store clerks or randomly on the Internet. There are many important things you need to know in order to create a targeted group of supplements for your individual needs. (These need-to-knows can be explained to you by your licensed healthcare practitioner or your *Fit, Fun and Fabulous* coach.)

* * *

Okay, now you know the basics of what your day in a *Fit, Fun and Fabulous* lifestyle will look like. Each of the following chapters will explain the importance of these lifestyle approaches. The biomarkers in the appendix will give you a clear understanding of the accelerated aging process—which this program will begin to reverse for you, if you are currently in that phase. If you are presently enjoying good health, your understanding of these biomarkers of aging will help you to avoid ever getting on the accelerated aging train. Mothers and fathers, please be aware that children can also experience this accelerated aging process, and increased numbers are suffering with the diseases of aging that previously were found only in adults, such as Type 2 diabetes and heart disease. Please champion this lifestyle for them so that they, too, can be *Fit, Fun and Fabulous* at any age.

This program will rejuvenate your biology on the cellular level, so get ready to reclaim your health and vitality. I ask you to commit to 12 weeks of this lifestyle and enjoy the same benefits that hundreds of my patients have received. Once you do that, I am convinced that you will want the *Fit, Fun and Fabulous* lifestyle to be your lifestyle for the rest of your life!

Below is the agreement to yourself and your current life assessment. Please complete them now as we begin the Fit Fun & Fabulous Program. After our first 12 weeks I will ask you to review your life assessment and recalculate your biological age. This is also a great time to revisit any blood test results your doctor may have been concerned with.

MY AGREEMENT

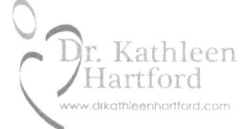

Right here and right now is where you will come to grips with one of the most important people in your life: YOU! Ask yourself: Am I ready, willing and able to make a commitment to myself and my future health by carrying out the assigned daily action plans within this Biological Rejuvenation Program? Keep in mind that from time to time you will compromise, and from time to time you will fail ... sometimes miserably. At times, the program won't work as fast as you had hoped, and some days it may feel as though it is not working at all.

Remember that this program is based in science. Healthy weight loss is a scientific formula, and improving your biological age is an outcome of this formula when applied as a committed lifestyle. So are you willing to stay the course? Remember, as humans we are imperfect, and it is in striving again and again that we succeed. Just stay the course.

Does this make sense to you? Will you participate in daily accountability and self-examination? If your response is "yes," you are on your way to personal change that includes not only biological rejuvenation but also personal growth and development.

You are now ready to sign your self-contract, your personal commitment to improving your health, revitalizing your life and knowing yourself in a deeper, more meaningful way.

NAME _____

DATE _____

> Note: *If you are unable to sign this commitment, it is possibly a sign of a deep wound or sabotaging pattern that prevents you from moving forward in your life. If this is the case, I ask that you take a few days to examine how being stuck or not having the ability to commit to a self-supportive process is at play in other areas of your life: your relationships, your eating, your career, your family. If you find that it is a common denominator in your life, then let's explore a way to change that. Sometimes an honest conversation with someone such as a close friend, spouse or a coach can help to work you through this pattern. Coaching is available through our office by visiting us on the web at* <drkathleenhartford.com> *or calling (800) 893-5000.*

MY LIFE ASSESSMENT

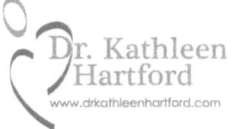

My experience with thousands of patients has
been that when we change the physical body, we
create change throughout the entire being. As you begin the *Fit, Fun and
Fabulous* program, I would like you to determine a baseline for how you
experience your life—maybe the better term is your "relation to your life."
To keep things simple and easy, this assessment is on a scale of 1 to 10.

10 = Perfect bliss and happiness in relation to this area

1 = Hopelessness and impending doom in this area

Instructions

Get out some paper and sit quietly. If you meditate, please enter that
meditative state. If you are not familiar with meditation then simply sit
upright in a comfortable chair, close your eyes, take a few deep breaths
and focus on the air moving into your body. Feel your lungs expanding
with the breath you take in, then gently release the air and feel your lungs
relaxing. As your lungs relax, your body and mind will relax. From this
peaceful state, be aware of your feelings about your life and rank each of
the following categories.

- **ETHICS**   _____

  Now there is a powerful word! You cannot be your best self and live
  a fulfilled life if you have no moral or ethical principles. Integrity is
  our ability to keep these principles; it is your code of honor or the
  wholeness of who you are. Living in integrity is vitally important for
  you to feel good about yourself on the inside. Ethics make you worth
  knowing. It is important to examine the ethical values that you base
  your day-to-day existence on. Creating a value-based life provides an
  inner sense of integrity and wholeness that nothing else can replace.

- **FAMILY**   _____

  Family is possibly the most important area, and also the one most
  commonly taken for granted. I continuously remind parents of the

importance and power they have in their children's lives. So many children are being raised by the media, the internet or their peers. They are being programmed to be people you would not be proud to have raised, and that is the question: Does your relationship with your children "raise them up" to match with your values-based life? Or does it leave them at the mercy of commercials, entertainers, friends and movie themes that are not in accord with what you say your household stands for? Children crave guidance and they will seek it out. Make sure it's your guidance that is on their radar screen and in their hearts. Teach them gentle and powerful lessons based on your values.

Relationships with parents, children and spouses are not only important to society and to you as an individual—they are the safe space where we should be able to 'land' for comfort and security at the end of the day. Can you imagine the world if everyone took care of their own, providing safety and support for each other? Can you imagine the type of family you could create if you became deeply interested in who your children and spouse are and then celebrated in that?

• FINANCES   _____

Now here is the American weakness. We have been trained to live above our means. Credit cards, credit lines, expensive toys ... they are all here for the taking. Yet I would venture to say that this area probably creates one of our greatest internal stressors. What if someone helped you to create a budget, set goals and held you to the task of getting out of debt? Social security will never allow you to live at your current level. In fact we cannot be guaranteed it will be available to us, because we have a government that also spends beyond it's means. As a responsible person, it is up to you to take care of yourself. Just as an athletic coach would never support an athlete in overindulging while in training, a personal coach would not allow you to over extend yourself financially. They would help you to first get out of debt, then budget for what you truly desire and make certain that personal time and family vacations are a part of that budget.

- **HEALTH** _____

  Everyone wants it, but few are willing to do what it takes to achieve and maintain it. I'm excited that by buying this book you are choosing to do just that! Let's be real, your body is the vehicle through which you will experience your life. If you were going on a cross-country trip, you wouldn't risk taking a broken-down vehicle. Yet we choose to live in broken-down bodies that might collapse at any moment. You will find it difficult to enjoy your life if you are racked with pain, unable to move, taking drugs to get through the day and living in a fog. As a coach, I am committed to you living your life FULL OUT, and you cannot do that with health challenges. Together, through the Fit Fun and Fabulous Program we will get your body in order so that you can get on with living your best life.

- **HOME** _____

  Home is where the heart is. What shape is your home in? Do you enter it and say, "Ah, thank God I'm home!" or do you walk in and say, "Oh my God, what a mess"? Your house is a reflection of you. Is it messy or anal-retentively tidy? Is it lived in? Is the furniture comfortable or is it there just for show? Your house is like your skin; you should be comfortable in it.

- **CAREER** _____

  Oftentimes, our work defines who we are. Have you ever asked yourself who you would be if you weren't a surgeon, a lawyer, a teacher or a homemaker? Do you know who you really are underneath the image you presently project? What would you like to do within your field? Do you want to continue to grow and learn in your current area or is there another area that you have always been interested in exploring?

- **EDUCATION** _____

  Have you always wanted to further your education? Are there certain conferences you should be attending to enhance your career? Would you like to begin to take unrelated classes in subjects you have always had an interest in? Perhaps you would like to study to be a better parent or improve your personal relationships or train your pet! Whatever interests you, knowledge is power and it can also be loads of fun. What are your educational goals?

- **RECREATION** _____

  Let's break down that word: re-create. This is where you get to recharge your batteries, pursue your passions and belly laugh. Recreation is vital to body, mind and spirit. It can be as simple as fishing, joining a gym or taking a dance class. Explore what brought you great joy as a child and do it! Chances are it will still be fun and you will feel like a new person when you're done.

- **SPIRITUAL** _____

  Do you believe in a power greater than you? If not, you probably spend a lot of time in fear. I do not care how you connect to spirit in your life, but research and experience shows that those who do are happier, healthier and live longer.

These are the important aspects that make up this incredible journey called your life. Awareness is the beginning of conscious living. Awareness of the above areas will give you a chance to explore where you are, who you are and how you want to be in the world. I will ask you to complete this section again at the end of 12 weeks. As stated above my experience is as you change your health on the inside it will create subtle changes in the other important areas of your life on the outside. Let this be the beginning:

Live your life with joy, purpose and passion!

Chapter 2

BIOLOGICAL AGE VERSUS CHRONOLOGICAL AGE

Who doesn't want to look and feel younger than their years? If the patients who come through my door are any indication, everyone does! The goal of this Biological Rejuvenation Program is to support you in becoming biologically younger this year than you were last year. In order to achieve this, you must first determine your current biological age.

Your Biological Age Assessment

Assessing your biological age is easy: visit <drkathleenhartford.com> and click on the *Biological Age Wheel* tab to create your biological age baseline. You are going to need your:

- Height and weight.
- Waist and hip measurements.
- Hand grip strength using a dynamometer. Perhaps your doctor or gym has one; if you don't have access to one, leave that blank and simply do push-ups. (The Biological Age Wheel allows you to use push-ups as a strength indicator.) If you are a guy, hit the floor with old-fashioned, plank-style push-ups; ladies can do a modified push-up on their knees if traditional push-ups are too difficult.

- Blood pressure (remember, the first number is the systolic pressure).
- Lean muscle mass and body fat percentage (most gyms can do this for you).

If possible, find a healthcare practitioner or a gym that has a bio-impedance instrument. Through bio-impedance analysis, you can determine not just your lean muscle mass, but also your water utilization level, cellular health and basal metabolic rate, along with toxicity and inflammatory indicators. Whenever water is being pushed outside of a cell rather than being maintained inside, this shows that an inflammatory condition is brewing. Your cell membrane permeability is also crucial and can be predicted through bio-impedance analysis. There are additional benefits to getting your body fat percentage and lean muscle mass percentage through bio-impedance verses a simple caliper test that pinches and measures fat on several areas of the body. If you are utilizing a different fat-measuring devise, such as a scale, please note that it will only provide the percentage of lower body fat as it measures leg to leg. If you are using a handheld instrument, it will only give you the measurement of upper body fat. I point this out because the percentage will be limited in actual body fat to a particular area; however, these numbers can still be used as a baseline to monitor the loss of body fat as you continue on the program. Just be aware that it is important to use the same fat-measuring device throughout the program, so that you are comparing apples to apples.

After you obtain the above information, we will use it to determine your:
- Muscle age
- Strength age
- Body fat age
- Body shape age
- Heart age

These indicators will be calculated by the *Biological Age Wheel* on <drkathleenhartford.com> to determine your biological age.

* * *

Congratulations! Were you surprised by the results? Whatever your initial biological age is, rest assured together, we can improve it!

Vital at Any Age

Getting older is a fact of life, but vitality and wellness are not only for the young. What's more, maturing into your adult years doesn't mean that you have to be riddled with aches and pains and disease. Throughout these pages, I will emphasize that your health is an accumulation of your choices. The food you eat, the liquids you drink, the thoughts you think, the words you say, the amount of rest and exercise you get—these daily actions and decisions are the building blocks that determine the quality of your life!

At the same time, it's possible that "you don't know what you don't know," and these unknowns can get you into trouble unless you become aware of them and educate yourself. For example, did you know that as you begin to lose fat pounds, organochlorine concentrations increase and suppress thyroid function? This suppression reduces T3—a very important thyroid hormone that supports additional fat loss—leaving you confused, frustrated and wondering why your fat loss has stalled. This is the time when many people give up on their continued weight loss and resort to their old destructive lifestyle habits.

There are ways to support the thyroid during weight loss so that you don't hit this frustrating fat loss stall (we will cover this on upcoming pages). This Biological Rejuvenation Program will make you aware of underlying factors that can have devastating effects on your health if left unchecked or unknown. Remember knowledge is power! By learning this information you will be able to make healthier lifestyle choices that will enhance your health each day.

Take my client Elaine, for example. She had become diabetic and was caught in a yo-yo cycle of weight gain and loss. Each time Elaine made serious progress, she eventually hit a plateau and became discouraged, she did not know about organochlorines or how to pull them from the system as they were released. With coaching and the Fit, Fun and Fabulous lifestyle approach, Elaine was able to lose 40 pounds of fat in 14 weeks and normalize her blood sugar from the 150-200 range down to the 80s!

A Definition of Biological Age

What is the significance of biological age versus chronological age? Your chronological age is simply your age in calendar years, and that age increases once a year when your birthday rolls around. Your biological age determines if your body is aging faster than your calendar years at the cellular level. The real difference, therefore, between your biological and chronological age is the health of your cells and their capacity to function at their highest level at any given time in your life. So, the question we are asking is: How does your biological age compare to your chronological age? Is it lower? It can be if you follow this program closely. You see, you can only be as healthy as your cells. The purpose of changing your biological age is to create healthier cells, which then translate into a physically-fit, more vibrant you. Your chronological age will continue to increase with each birthday. My wish is for you to have lots of birthdays, but I also wish for you to feel good each time a birthday rolls around. This is YOUR life and my goal is to ensure that it is filled with *vitality!*

Now that you know the difference between your biological age and chronological age, you can become more powerful in creating optimal health in your body and, ultimately, your life. My guess is that your biological age is close to your chronological age. By working with this Biological Rejuvenation Program, let's see if we can make you biologically younger than your years.

How Your Biological Age Indicators Correlate to the 12 Biomarkers of Aging

Biological age indicators (which you just calculated, to determine your biological age) are a window into how your body is aging. Researchers at Tufts University have determined that certain ages have certain markers; if we can keep our markers below the average age marker for our chronological age, we can maintain our youth on a biological or cellular level. If we find that our biological indicators are higher than the average indicators for our chronological age, we know that we are on the road to accelerated aging, disease and possibly early death. If nothing else, we will not have the vibrancy and energy that allow us to enjoy life through our physical body as we age.

Personal Power Comes from Personal Responsibility

I am hoping that you will explore the *12 Biomarkers of Aging* in detail. (I have placed them in the Appendix as a reference because I know that the Type A personalities out there just want me to get on with telling you what you can do in your life to recapture or maintain your biological youth!) I believe that information is power; it gives you the opportunity to be self-responsible—being able to respond and act for yourself. The truth is that everything in our environment is "information" being given to some aspect of your body. Here are a few examples: If you walk into a cold room, the temperature gives your body information and it responds by creating goose bumps to conserve body heat; when you lift weights, the stress on your muscles is information that tells those muscles to build up more muscle tissue to manage this stress; when you drink a cup of coffee, the information is telling your body to jumpstart the adrenal gland; when you sit in meditation and focus on your breathing, the information is telling your body and mind to slow down; when the person you dated doesn't call the next day, the information is that he or she isn't interested. So you see, we take information in on every level of our conscious and subconscious being. When we choose to not be aware of this information flow, we lose our power.

Many of the problems with our nation's healthcare system are the consequence of giving others power over us. The old paradigm of healthcare (which is still prevalent today) was to treat your body like your car: wait until it breaks down then go to a doctor to fix it. Even when medicine promotes early detection, you still have it! You have not prevented anything you simply found it sooner. The truth is that, unlike your car, your body has an innate intelligence that made it, maintains it and keeps it striving for health every day. Think about it. Your body can take a peanut butter and jelly sandwich and make new eye cells; really, do you know a scientist who can do that? Your body can take two cells from two different people and make a new human being. Even more amazing is that this new being is -perfectly formed with all its parts functioning after 12 short weeks—and it's only the size of your little finger. Absolutely amazing! When I was carrying my daughter, I never had to think, *Oh we are making liver cells today so I had better do …* No, the body (through this amazing innate intelligence) just did it while I was riding my horse, climbing mountains or eating an apple! Your body is powerful and will last for a hundred years provided there is no interference to that innate intelligence, AND you give it the raw materials required to maintain itself and make healthy new cells.

Believe me, there are many people in the world who would be more than happy to run your life and take your power away from you—the government, pharmaceutical companies, perhaps even your family—but the people I know who are vibrant and full of life have little to do with being controlled by others, especially when it comes to their health. Personal power comes from personal responsibility. Remember, the biomarkers of aging are in the realm of science; they are definable and reversible and, therefore, within your control. Now that you have this information, your ability to respond is heightened. Let's be powerful together!

Chapter 3

HEALTHY EATING AND EATING FREQUENCY

9 mentioned this earlier, but it bears repeating: your life is truly the sum total of your choices. The quality of your days is created through the food you eat, the thoughts you think, the air you breath, the water you drink, the environment you live in, even the dietary supplements you take and your ability to eliminate biological waste. True, some aspects of our lives—such as the air or our work environment—may be difficult to control, but in most areas of our lives we do have the direct ability to make choices every day. These are the areas that I'd like you to think about as you read through this book and begin to apply its principles.

My client Cynthia, for example, had an enormous amount of stress in her job and was eight years older biologically than her chronological age of 55. She came to my office complaining of neck, shoulder, arm and hand pain, dizziness, depression, weight gain and irregular bowel movements. Determined to manage the aspects of her life that she could control, Cyndi made the decision to work with one of our personal trainers. We set her up with exercise and the Fit Fun & Fabulous program including medical foods to help manage environmental stressors (more on that in an upcoming chapter). Cyndi has since lost 19 pounds of fat and regained 12 years of her biological youth!

Healthy Eating

We will now discuss three very important points in regards to healthy eating: anti-inflammatory foods, the glycemic index of foods and how to balance acid and alkaline (ash) foods. By the end of this chapter, you will see how easy and common-sense-based this approach is.

Before we get to those three points, however, the first health-enhancing lifestyle habit I'd like to explore with you is the frequency with which you eat. Healthy eating and eating frequency go hand in hand and are equally important in being able to sustain healthy cells.

"How and what should I eat?" This has always been my favorite area of discussion with my patients. Many will schedule an initial appointment with me to review their diet and to learn how they can eat correctly. They want to feel better and to lose weight, both of which are very good goals. The truth is that I can outline what they need to do to achieve this in the first ten minutes of our hour-long consult. This is what I tell them:

1. **Eat food the way God made it—the way it grows naturally on the earth—and avoid genetically modified foods (GMO) at all costs.** The optimal diet to enjoy is a plant-based diet: mostly fruits and vegetables with limited grains and, light forms of protein as outlined in your *Anti-inflammatory Food Schedule* (in the Appendix). As much as possible, choose organic food in order to avoid all of the pesticides, herbicides and pharmaceuticals that are released into our environment or fed directly to our food supply.

This is a serious matter. According to the pollution information website (scorecard.org), more than four billion pounds of toxic industrial chemicals are released into the nation's environment each year, including 72 million pounds of recognized carcinogens. Industrial facilities alone dump 232 million pounds of toxic chemicals into America's waterways. FOX News reported on April 20, 2009, that 271 million pounds of pharmaceuticals have been released into our nation's waterways. What's more, exposure to growth hormones in beef could be putting Americans at risk for infertility. A recent study found that women who routinely ate beef were far more likely to give birth to boys who grow up to have lower-than-normal sperm counts. Hormone residues in beef have been implicated in the early onset of puberty in girls, which could put them at greater risk of developing breast and other forms of cancer.

2. **Avoid processed food.** Companies that produce processed food (using the term loosely) do not, and never will, know as much about your body as the Creator who created it. To clarify these choices further, please refer to the *Anti-inflammatory Food Schedule* in the Appendix. This list of food is very important because you will want to quiet inflammation in the gut and throughout the body.

In the previous chapter, we discussed biological age versus chronological age and how the accelerated aging process begins in the body. The thing to remember is this: accelerated aging and most disease processes begin with inflammation. In today's post-modern world, we are inundated with various environmental toxins and pharmaceuticals such as steroids, antibiotics and birth control pills that affect the body, slowly but surely breaking down the digestive system and disrupting the balance of flora in the intestinal tract.

Sadly, on top of this, we feed ourselves, and our children, nutrient-sparse, high-sugar foods that feed the Candida albicans or what is commonly referred to as yeast in the digestive system. This further contributes to an imbalance of gut flora and ultimately a penetration of the intestinal wall. Once these delicate systems are compromised, they lose their ability to digest and absorb food correctly or to act as a barrier to food particles that are not meant to penetrate through the intestinal wall. This compromise of the intestinal wall allows the introduction into the blood stream of many substances, which may be antigenic. These constant assaults on the body lead to most of our allergies, which oftentimes lead to childhood and adult asthma, chronic immune dysfunction and, more recently, new immune diseases such as chronic fatigue and fibromyalgia. Children who come into my chiropractic office are usually there because of chronic immune challenges, not for back and neck pain. Trust me, their parents are coming to me as a last resort after having been on the antibiotic merry-go-round with continuously recurring illnesses.

In older children and adults this compromised intestinal tract has been associated with depression, anxiety, recurring irritability, heartburn, indigestion, lethargy, extreme food and environmental allergies, acne, migraine headaches, reoccurring cystitis, or vaginal infections, premenstrual tension, or menstrual problems. Unfortunately their medical doctor often tells them that they are suffering from "neurotic anxiety syndrome" or depression and are given inappropriate medications, which further exacerbate their condition. If you review the list above you will see that none of the conditions have been identified with any disease entity they are simply an outcome of a compromised gut, which creates a compromised immune response.

The following scenario is an example of a typical conversation when adult patients come to my office complaining of chronic issues, such as fibromyalgia, chronic fatigue, gastric reflux, constipation, migraines, respiratory system weakness, exhaustion and many forms of depression:

> *Question:* So tell me about your childhood. Were you sick often or does one illness stand out in your mind?
>
> *Patient:* Well, I did have ear infections a lot growing up ... or ... I did get strep throat as a child ... or ... once I was hospitalized for pneumonia and now I get bronchitis, colds or the flu every year.
>
> *Question:* So you have had several courses of antibiotics?
>
> *Patient:* Well, yes.
>
> *Question:* Did you ever reinstate the good bacteria in your digestive tract?
>
> *Patient:* I eat yogurt. Doesn't that count? The TV commercials make it sound like it works!
>
> *Answer:* That's not enough. You need several different colonies in the tens of billions to balance and restore the lost colonies of good bacteria in the intestinal tract.

In my professional experience, a compromised intestinal tract begins with childhood ear infections or sore throats for which medical doctors—following proper medical protocol—prescribe antibiotics. The child then develops food or environmental allergies, which oftentimes lead to asthmatic attacks—especially while playing soccer, football, running track or during the change of seasons. When an attack happens, they are given a steroid inhaler, which further supports the feeding of yeast in the system and further compromises the intestinal tract. Sometimes children will appear to outgrow these conditions, but usually they develop into something else, such as adult immune challenges, digestive issues and chronic or recurring diseases.

To begin the healing process, we must go back to the beginning: the imbalance created in the intestinal tract, (or gut)—which, by the way, houses approximately 76 percent of your immune system—and its corresponding inflammatory state. We do this by eating low-inflammatory foods—in other words, foods that are not going to irritate the gut while we support the healing of the intestinal lining and reinstate the good bacteria that have been lost over the years due to well-intentioned medications. (We will address how to restore gut flora with targeted nutrients in a later chapter).

While you are following this Biological Rejuvenation Program, I will ask you to count your daily food choices on the *Anti-inflammatory Food Schedule* in the Appendix. (This schedule is also included for your convenience in the *Fit, Fun and Fabulous Journal.*) On one side of that page are foods that you can enjoy; have as much of them as you'd like. On the other side of the page are foods to avoid; these are the high inflammatory gut-irritating foods that will diminish your overall health while increasing body fat, producing mucus, creating acidity in the system and, in the case of low-quality carbohydrates, contributing to insulin resistance.

At the same time, there is another very important index to consider. Go to your computer and do a search for "glycemic index" or "GI foods." You will find an enormous amount of information on the importance of maintaining healthy blood sugar levels and how food directly affects these levels.

Look at the foods listed on the *Glycemic Index* in the Appendix and let's review some basics. There are high-glycemic index foods and low-glycemic index foods. Low-glycemic index foods help to maintain normal blood sugar levels. High-glycemic index foods contribute to insulin resistance, which as you now know is the first step towards accelerated aging and potentially serious health complications such as diabetes and heart disease. Examples of low-glycemic foods are brown rice, healthy proteins, vegetables, apples, barley, grapefruit, legumes, nuts, oatmeal, green peas, tomatoes and unsweetened (and ideally, organic) yogurt. Examples of high-glycemic foods are (as you may have guessed) white rice, white bread, sweet snacks, sodas, cereal, chips and white potatoes. Most of these high-glycemic foods have little to no nutrient value and the body burns them very quickly. They contribute to inflammation, insulin resistance, obesity and disease. Low-glycemic foods are also very high in fiber content, while high-glycemic foods are low in fiber and high in sugar. Fiber feeds the vitally important good bacteria in your gut, while simple sugars feed the inappropriate bacteria and yeast.

So, what's the healthiest thing you can do for your body right here, right now? Balance your blood sugar by choosing low-glycemic, anti-inflammatory food. This is not just a problem unique to diabetics. Remember, you are not born a Type 2 diabetic; you become Type 2 diabetic through poor lifestyle choices;

Take the case of my client Diane. At age 60, Diane came to my office 80-plus pounds overweight and on a downward spiral with Type 2 diabetes.

"I've been a compulsive eater and yo-yo dieter my entire life," Diane shared. *"I can't remember the last time I was on the minus side of 200 pounds. I'm disheartened!"*

Diane also suffered from high blood pressure, poor sleep patterns, low energy and had been treated for uterine cancer. When I presented the Fit, Fun and Fabulous program, she was skeptical because she had tried every diet known to man. Midway through the program, Diane had recovered seven years of her biological youth, lost 41 pounds of inflammatory fat tissue and was at her lightest weight since 1989. Most importantly, her medical doctor was able to reduce her diabetic medication since her A1C glycated hemoglobin (which reflects your average blood sugar levels over a two- to three-month period) decreased from 8.0 to 6.4 (with normal being 4 to 5.9) ... and the program was effective at eliminating the Dawn phenomenon—the nighttime blood sugar spikes that so many diabetics struggle with.

Sadly, it's not just adults who struggle with Type 2 diabetes (originally called adult onset diabetes). The American Diabetic Association predicts that one-third of today's children will suffer from Type 2 diabetes, *a completely preventable disease* that can lead to the loss of kidney function, loss of eyesight and sometimes the amputation of limbs as the sugar destroys the circulatory system.

Currently, 21 million Americans are living with diabetes, and another 54 million are living with pre-diabetes or metabolic syndrome. The American Diabetes Association reports that diabetes costs Americans $174 billion per year. At the same time, it is estimated that 91 percent of diabetic cases are lifestyle-related, largely driven by widespread obesity and therefore preventable.

As a parent, if you were giving your child daily doses of a poison that created a debilitating disease, you would be arrested and charged with child abuse, and rightfully so. Yet for whatever reason, our country allows large corporations and fast food franchises to produce food that has been scientifically proven to destroy our children's health; worse yet, parents give into these marketing ploys and their children's demands, pretending that a little poison doesn't matter. The good news is that you now know that it does matter—at any age—and you can begin to makes changes in your family's diet that will have lifelong benefits for your own health and the health of your family.

Eating Frequency

This brings me to the second part of this chapter's topic: eating frequency. I strongly advise you to begin eating five times daily: three main meals and two smaller snacks. Also, consider reducing your portion sizes. This point was visually brought home to me the other day when I pulled out my grandmother's china for a family dinner I was having. Her dinner plates were about two-thirds the size of the plates I use today—so, begin taking smaller portions or just eating from smaller plates! This alone could cut down your caloric intake by about one-third with very little effort.

The reason for the small snacks is actually twofold: they help stabilize and regulate your blood sugar levels and will prevent you from being so hungry at your next meal that you empty the refrigerator before you sit down at the table. Obviously, this will help you tremendously if you are trying to decrease your fat percentage, increase your lean muscle mass and generally create a healthier body. A healthy snack could be a handful of nuts, an apple or organic yogurt with fruit. Keeping it light but nourishing is the key to a fabulous life!

Whatever you do, don't skip a meal. Skipping meals will decrease your basal metabolic rate and increase your deposits of fat. It will also send a signal to your body that you need to metabolize (or, break down to use as fuel) your own muscle tissue—yes, muscle tissue—to maintain healthy blood sugar levels. Do an online search for "gluconeogenesis" or read about the *12 Biomarkers of Aging* (in the Appendix) and you will learn why this is the most expedient way for your body to create necessary sugar/fuel when no glucose is present in the system—something you definitely don't want your body to do.

Finally, I would like to reiterate how the food on your plate should look to balance your pH (your alkaline versus acidic food). Acidic foods are proteins (mostly meats), processed carbohydrates and sweets; the last two we are trying to avoid. Alkaline foods are fruits and vegetables. So if you look at your plate, one-third of it should be filled with "acid ash" foods of your choosing. If you are a meat eater choose an organic high-quality protein about the size of the palm of your hand. A big person has a larger hand and requires more protein; a smaller person has a smaller hand and requires less protein. The rest of your plate should be filled with vegetables. Enjoy your fruits separately. If you do only that for your main meals, you will be amazed at how much more energy you have and how much easier it will be to lose weight—and you won't ever have to wonder again about what you should eat.

* * *

To recap the topics in this chapter and how simple they are:

Eat healthy nutrient-dense food the way it comes from the earth. Have one-third of the food on your plate be acid ash in the form of protein—preferably organic, from an animal or plant source—and two-thirds be alkaline food from vegetables. Enjoy a multitude of colors in your vegetables and low-glycemic starch selections.

Eat frequently, preferably five times a day—two of which can be small snacks to help stabilize your blood sugar levels and control hunger cravings.

Pretty easy, right? *Buon appetito!*

Chapter 4

THE PERILS OF
METABOLIC SYNDROME

*Y*ou now know the importance of making healthy food choices and eating frequently in a balanced fashion, but what are the consequences of making unhealthy food choices and regularly skipping meals? At the very least, we make ourselves vulnerable to metabolic syndrome, also referred to as syndrome X or insulin resistance. (For more information on this, see *Biomarker 5: Body Fat Distribution* and *Biomarker 7: Blood Sugar Tolerance*, in the Appendix). People with metabolic syndrome are at increased risk of coronary heart disease, stroke, peripheral vascular disease and Type 2 diabetes.

Metabolic syndrome has become increasingly common in the United States; an estimated 80 million Americans have it. This syndrome is characterized by a group of metabolic risk factors that occur in a person. They include:

- Abdominal obesity (excessive fat tissue in and around the abdomen)
- High blood fats, high triglycerides and high LDL cholesterol
- Low HDL cholesterol
- Elevated blood pressure

- Insulin resistance or glucose intolerance (the body can't properly use insulin or blood sugar)
- Pro-inflammatory state (for example, chronic pain or elevated C-reactive protein in the blood)
- Waist measuring 40 inches or more for men, and 35 inches or more for women

The dominant underlying risk factors for this syndrome appear to be abdominal obesity and insulin resistance. Insulin resistance is a generalized metabolic disorder in which the body can't use insulin efficiently as the cell wall becomes resistant to insulin released by the pancreas. (This is why metabolic syndrome is also called insulin resistance syndrome.) Initially, symptoms may include common things such as feeling sluggish after eating, experiencing dull headaches related to certain foods and excess weight gain, especially around the abdomen. These symptoms are created by the dysregulation of blood sugar levels and can ultimately lead to obesity, low blood sugar (hypoglycemia) and high blood sugar (hyperglycemia) fluctuations, high blood pressure, insulin resistance, high blood fats and, worst of all, Type 2 diabetes.

America has the fastest growing adolescent population of Type 2 diabetics, which is largely driven by obesity. Clearly, obesity is on the increase with our children; an estimated 16 to 33 percent of children in the United States are obese, and 60 percent of adults are overweight or obese—totaling 108 million people. It's not difficult to figure out why childhood obesity has become a national epidemic. Youngsters spend sedentary hours each day in front of TVs, video games and computers. Schools either no longer require or have greatly reduced physical education classes, and potentially dangerous streets keep our kids inside rather than outdoors playing sports and exercising. Coupled with the proliferation of fast food and sugar-laden snacks, our children's bodies are facing even greater challenges.

One major obstacle to children's health is the easy availability of zero-nutrient beverages such as carbonated sodas, sweetened juices and caffeine-laden "sports" drinks. According to a recent study published in *The Lancet*, a leading medical journal in the United Kingdom, children who consume these beverages are at a greater risk for developing obesity. If you are a parent of young children, it's important to know that a recent Harvard University study concluded that the odds of becoming obese increases 1.6 times for every can, bottle or glass of sugary beverage consumed daily. Remember it has been determined that one-third of our children—and please pay attention to this—born since the year 2000 will become diabetic.

Also remember that diabetes is a horrible disease accounting for nearly 73,000 deaths in America alone and with the potential and probable long-term ramifications being loss of sensation, eyesight, stroke, heart disease and at times amputation of limbs and kidney failure. (See biomarker #7 in the appendix for information on the connection between Diabetes and Alzheimer's disease) This is not a disease that we, as good parents, intentionally inflict upon our children. When we don't take control of the dietary habits within our own households, however, we leave not only ourselves but our children vulnerable to this disease and other hazards of accelerated aging. The difference between our generation and younger generations is that their aging process will be so severely accelerated that they are estimated to be the first generation that will not live as long as their parents. Is this really the legacy that we wish to leave for our children—an inheritance of disease and early death?

Start by Making Simple Changes

You can begin to avoid falling prey to these daunting statistics by taking some simple actions. First, remember that in your own home you determine the quality of food and drinks that everyone consumes. Instead of having sugary beverages in the kitchen, offer filtered water to your family. When your children are thirsty, they will drink what is available, and if only water is available, that is what they will reach for. Have some bowls of chopped carrots, celery, broccoli or whole fruit on the counter and you will be amazed at the little fingers that will grab it each time they walk by. Try it ... it really does work, and soon your child's taste buds will be programmed to enjoy healthy food. (By the way, this works for the adults in the house, as well.)

I find it interesting when I hear parents say that their child will not eat vegetables or will only drink soda. It amazes me because I have yet to see a three-year-old jump in the car and go to the store to buy his or her groceries! As adults, it is our job to set an example for our children. They may be little people, but just like all other humans, children's bodies are designed to eat when they are hungry and drink when they are thirsty. Our job is to ensure that they have healthy foods within easy reach whenever they are hungry or thirsty.

When it comes to fluids, aim for a daily formula of two-thirds of an ounce of water for every pound of body weight; in other words, take .66 times your current body weight and you will know the exact amount of water (in ounces) that your body requires. If you live in a dry environment or exercise intensely, you may require more. If you are on a fluid-restricted diet, I suggest that you speak to your doctor about this.

It is important to make sure the quality of the water you drink is clean and pure. Recently while traveling with my mother, I was purchasing high-quality filtered water when she said to me, "You know, Kath, we live in America. You can drink the water." I laughed because I begged to differ. In fact, several times a year I give presentations about the devastating effects of environmental toxins on our health. According to the Centers For Disease Control (CDC), perchlorate (a solid rocket fuel chemical that interferes with thyroid and brain development in children) has been found in our water. Pharmaceuticals that we flush or eliminate through our urine also end up in our drinking water, not to mention fluoride and a host of other pollutants. Trust me, America's water supply is not as safe as you may like to believe.

You can, in moderation, mix things up with limited amounts of fruit juice. Keep in mind that it takes approximately five apples to make a glass of apple juice. How long would it take you to eat five apples? Quite a long time, and you would be getting all of the natural fiber that the Creator put in there to slow down that blood sugar absorption. On the other hand, it takes only minutes to drink the glass of juice. We no longer have the fiber present, and it will spike our blood sugar. (Remember, spiking blood sugar is what begins the downward spiral of insulin resistance.) My suggestion is that you dilute your fruit juices with an equal amount of water and have it as a treat.

Unfortunately, even healthy drinks such as green tea do not substitute for our necessary water intake. They are good and have health benefits, but only water is water, so enjoy it abundantly. I always tell my patients, "If you wouldn't shower in it to clean your body on the outside, don't expect it to clean your body on the inside." Adding lemon or slices of fruit to your water can enhance its flavor, and it looks so refreshing. Lemon has an extra cleansing benefit, as well.

When Jim, 55, entered our office, he was a broken man— depressed, anxious, moody and unable to sleep. He was overweight, constantly fatigued and suffered from pain in his chest, muscles and joints. Jim had all of signs of metabolic syndrome: high cholesterol, high blood pressure, and an unhealthy waist-to-hip ratio. He had already had a heart attack and two stents, and was taking multiple medications—from Neurotin to Lipitor to Vicodin. If we didn't get Jim's metabolic syndrome under control, his future health picture would be grim.

Jim began the Fit, Fun and Fabulous program weighing 238 pounds; his body fat percentage was 25.7, or 65.8 pounds of fat, which is essentially inflammatory tissue. Less than a month into the program, Jim had 18 pounds of weight loss, some of which was water weight due to the toxicity load on his body, but nine pounds of which was fat. Within nine months, he had lost 47 pounds—nearly 20 pounds of it was fat tissue—and was down to 23 percent body fat. Jim's intracellular water now exceeded his extracellular water, indicating a great decrease in toxicity. But most importantly, Jim was feeling young again. He was able to begin exercising regularly with very little discomfort. Now, Jim has much more energy and vitality than he ever thought possible. Looking back, he clearly sees how metabolic syndrome was stealing his good health.

To recap the perils of metabolic syndrome, it is characterized by the following indicators, which accelerate the aging process:

- High blood pressure
- Abnormal cholesterol metabolism

- High triglycerides
- High insulin levels
- Increased body fat
- Increased waist-to-hip ratio
- Decreased muscle mass
- Decreased strength

You can begin today to make better choices with your food, drinks and the frequency of your meals that will work towards balancing your blood sugar, thereby moving you away from metabolic syndrome ... not just for yourself, but also for those you love.

Chapter 5

LIFE IS MOTION

Did you know that motion is vital for all functions of the body? In fact, it is so important that I'm devoting this entire chapter to exploring how the biomechanical aspect of motion impacts our health and vitality.

With so much movement going on with the body all the time, it is not an exaggeration to say; "life is motion." From the molecular vibrations to the (e)motional expressions, motion affects us down to the very core our being. One of the most obvious "movements" that our bodies partake in is the daily ritual of going to the bathroom. In order to be healthy, we must efficiently eliminate waste products from the body. The body's circulatory and lymphatic systems also benefit from movement. Movement even affects—through the hormonal system—our moods and outlook on life.

It is really exciting to understand the dynamics of the body in motion—indeed it is quite "dynamic!" When I say "life is motion," I literally mean that everything about our bodies and the world we inhabit is continuously in motion. We live in a vibrating universe comprised of swirling molecules that come together to create matter. Our bodies are part of that matter.

In the very near future, I believe that science will understand more about the importance of vibration, especially in the area of vibrational medicine. Science always lags behind clinical experience because science is limited by its current technology. In other words, science cannot prove something that it does not yet have the tools to prove. Homeopathy, acupuncture, flower remedies and color therapy are just a few of the vibrational healing modalities that have been around for hundreds and (in the case of acupuncture) thousands of years; I use them in my practice daily with outstanding results. There are many good books available to explain vibrational healing, but I would suggest that you begin with *Power versus Force* and *Healing and Recovery*, both by Dr. David R. Hawkins, and *The Healing Power of Water* by Masaru Emoto, as you read this book remember that your body is comprised of approximately 70% water.

Whether it is the vibration of your thoughts, the food you eat or the company you keep, vibration determines your congruency with what is taking place in and around you—and your level of congruency determines your outcomes. In my daily work with patients, I find that all of these things are intimately connected. For more insights on this subject, visit my *Ramblings Of a Mad Woman* blog at <drkathleenhartford.com>.

For the moment, let's address the biomechanical movement of the body. Remember the lyrics to that old song: "The foot bone's connected to the anklebone / the anklebone's connected to the leg bone / the leg bone's connected to the knee bone"? This is all true! And because of this connection, when we ask one area of the body to move, it affects every other area—from our bones to our organs. When we look at the musculoskeletal body, we must look at it as joints in motion, intricately connected and balanced with each other through a network of nerves that is so complex, science cannot begin to replicate it. One step takes the coordination of more than 200 muscles (yes, one step!). Your jaw balances with your pelvis, and a misaligned pelvis can begin a degenerative process in your knee. The curves in your neck will affect the curves and discs of your low back; when your neck is misaligned for years, your soft discs will begin to bulge and degenerate not only in the neck area but also in your low back. This is due to the stress of incorrect gravitational forces on the lumbar (low back) vertebrae. Much of the low back pain I see in my office actually began with a reversal of the natural curve in the neck. If the neck loses its normal forward curve, or "lordosis," it can also create knifelike pain between the shoulder blades as it forces that curve to compensate for the misalignment above it. Remember, your body is always responding to information, and everything you do, think and speak is information for your body—even the position of your skeleton.

Why Chiropractic Care is Necessary for Good Health

Living in your body does not have to be painful. Our joints are meant to support us throughout our lives. When you experience joint pain, it is your body speaking to you about an imbalance. As a chiropractor, I am always interested in prevention, so let's review how we create misalignments that lead to imbalances—not just in our musculoskeletal system, but also in the central nervous system (our body's main communication system).

The purpose of the central nervous system is to coordinate every cell, tissue and organ in the body. This is why seemingly miraculous cures happen with people under chiropractic care. From ear infections to terminal illnesses, every chiropractor has experienced these miracles in their offices, and my guess is you have also heard of a few, because chiropractic is possibly the most effective tool available to normalize the central nervous system's function. So if a condition (from pain to an organ dysfunction) is related to interference with the central nervous system's ability to communicate and the chiropractic correction removes that interference, then the problem will usually resolve, oftentimes immediately. Clearly, chiropractic does not heal pain, terminal illness or infections, but it can help normalize the body's central nervous system function so that the body can do its job unimpeded. Only the body can heal itself; a chiropractor's job is to remove any interference to that healing process through the chiropractic adjustment.

A chiropractic adjustment on its own can and will produce miracles. When combined with therapeutic approaches that balance the five aspects of health, function is restored, nutrients are available, emotions are balanced and the body will have all that it needs to do its job of healing.

Misalignments of the cranium, spine and pelvis usually begin with trauma, physical, emotional or toxic. Oftentimes, the first trauma occurs during the birth process only to be followed by childhood falls, sports injuries, toxicity, severe emotional events or general stress. I see it all the time: a child falls and hits his head, cries but eventually stops—so the parent doesn't look into the situation any further. Or, a mother comes to my office following a car accident, but leaves her child at home because he isn't complaining of the same whiplash pain that is debilitating her. The child may never complain of the same pain but the child's immune system may begin to struggle, or the child may begin getting headaches, seizures or a whole host of maladies that are seemingly unrelated to the traumatic accident. Pain comes with degeneration. Degeneration occurs over time and medical doctors refer to it as arthritis. Arthritis will always develop in the area of injury that created misalignment to the spine if it has been left uncorrected. I spend a good part of my day explaining to parents the importance of wellness and preventative care for their children, so that they do not suffer with pain, headaches, muscle spasms and debilitation of movement down the road.

My own daughter was hit in the head with a basketball while in gym class at age 14, but she knew enough to ask the school nurse to call me. Her neck muscles were beginning to spasm and her shoulders were high and rolled forward. We did an assessment and found that her cervical/ neck curve had a complete reversal. Her body would have adapted to the loss of normal neck positioning within 72 hours or so, and she would have probably forgotten that hit on the head. If the incident had gone unchecked, the chances are quite good that after a few months she would have started getting severe headaches and, because of her age, she probably would have been told that the headaches were hormone-related. Possibly she would have been advised to go on to birth control pills—

which have their own complications. Eventually she would have lost her healthy posture, with her shoulders rounding forward to compensate for the forward head carriage. Perhaps one day in her 30s, 40s or 50s, while making her bed or exercising or sneezing, she would have moved a bit oddly and, with her spine in such a compensated posture, her discs would not be able to take the pressure any longer and ... bingo! ... she would have an acute bulging disc. Possible back surgery, chronic back pain, headaches and potential reproductive cancers would have been her future.

I'm certain that you know of someone who has a similar story—maybe it is you. If a person eventually sees a doctor of chiropractic for the back pain, that person might be told something like: "It looks as though you have an old injury to your neck, I can identify this because there are more arthritic changes there than anywhere else in your spine. Were you in an auto accident 15 or 20 years ago?" (Yes, the degeneration/arthritic changes will indicate when it happened.) Maybe the person would say, "No, no accidents." This is when I ask the patient to go home and check with his or her mother (mothers remember everything!). Baby walkers rolling down the stairs and coming to an abrupt stop at the bottom, falls from trees, hits in the head by a sibling, even hit by a car ... these types of accidents have been forgotten by my patients, but recalled by their mothers when asked.

This is 'just the stuff that life is made of'. Falls and accidents occur every day. While in school, we are educated and even required to have our eyes, ears and teeth checked, and as adults we are encouraged to get annual physicals. For some reason, however, when it comes to the spinal structure that supports every movement we make and houses the delicate nervous system responsible for communicating with every cell tissue and organ in our body, chiropractic spinal exams not only aren't required ... they are often times discouraged. This allows our spine to degenerate until we can no longer stand up straight or manage the pain that comes from its degeneration.

At this point, you are probably wondering why your primary care physician has never suggested that you have your child's spine examined.

Well, here's why: In 1987, a judge named Getzendanner agreed that there was a conspiracy (which had been active for decades) by the American Medical Association to eliminate the chiropractic profession. They engaged in educating doctors and patients that chiropractors were quacks, occult-like and uneducated. The truth is that chiropractic is a philosophy, science and an art that requires no less than 4,200 hours of chiropractic education with a minimum 1,000 hours of supervised clinical training. Chiropractors must have passed their national boards and a state board of examination, and then return for continuing education each year that they practice. People tend to trust their medical doctors to determine if they need a chiropractor, but the truth is that your medical doctor would require an additional 2,200 hours of education to practice chiropractic himself. This is why chiropractors are licensed primary care providers and require no referral from a medical doctor. The effectiveness of chiropractic procedures is why most insurance companies, including automobile and workman's compensation, cover chiropractic care. In fact, for the following reasons, I would make certain that you choose a policy that has this benefit.

According to the *Archives Of Internal Medicine*, of the seven million insurance members with chiropractic coverage versus one million who did not, the chiropractic members had:

- 37 percent fewer image tests
- 41 percent fewer hospitalizations
- 32 percent fewer back surgeries
- 28 percent overall reduction in the cost of treatment

The reason that the American Medical Association was not successful at destroying the chiropractic profession with their restraint of trade practices is because chiropractic is so effective that people demand it.[1]

---

1   On September 25, 1987, Getzendanner issued her opinion that the AMA had violated Section 1, but not 2, of the Sherman Act, and that it had engaged in an unlawful conspiracy in restraint of trade "to contain and eliminate the chiropractic profession" (Wilk v. AMA, 1987). She further opined that the "AMA had entered into a long history of illegal behavior," and then issued a permanent injunction against the AMA under Section 16 of the Clayton Act to prevent such future behavior.

I am thinking now of my client Kim. At age 57, she came to my office as a basic chiropractic patient with neck, shoulder and arm pain, and tingling in her hands and fingertips. She also had lower back stiffness, knee pain and foot pain. Kim's spinal structure was obviously challenged, creating gravitational stress to the joints of her extremities, along with pressure on her nervous system—hence, the tingling. I would like to use Kim's story as a teachable moment. Consider this: if there was enough stress on the nervous system to cause sensory pain in the shoulder, arm and hand, what do you think might be happening to the non-sensory fibers of the nervous system as it struggles to communicate information to every cell tissue and organ in the body? That analogy illustrates the importance of chiropractic for a body's overall ability to function at its highest level. Said another way, could you imagine reading this book or having a conversation when only partial information, perhaps every third word, was available? How effective do you think that would be? The same hold true for your body; to be healthy, it must receive all neurological information as it travels from the brain to the spinal cord, through the 24 movable bones of your spine as your spine works to keep you upright and active. Combine the neurological importance of this with the weight-bearing gravitational forces as they translate through your joints and create balance in your muscles, and you will understand why it's difficult to imagine how anyone could live a vital, active life without chiropractic care!

Okay, back to Kim. She understood the importance of chiropractic care, but she also knew that the pain she was experiencing was exacerbated by inflammation, due to excessive body fat. So Kim started the Fit, Fun and Fabulous program and lost 14 pounds—11 of which were inflammatory fat. She also recovered seven years of biological youth! Of course her tingling and pain resolved completely.

No matter what physical shape a person is in, I recommend that everyone have a spinal assessment by a licensed doctor of chiropractic. Ask your friends and family for a referral; you will be surprised to discover how many have a chiropractor that they love and trust. Schedule an appointment and give yourself the greatest possible chance of maintaining healthy joints, healthy motion and a healthy central nervous system throughout your life.

The Spine is in Constant Motion

The dynamic nature of the spine allows for balance through continuous adaptation to positions, restrictions and gravitational forces. You now know that incorrect alignment can affect the muscles, tendons and ligaments around a joint, the discs or soft tissue between a joint—and, most importantly, the nerve information exiting from the spinal cord between the spinal bones. This intimate balancing affects more than just the spine. A very elementary example might be if your pelvis is misaligned or you have rotation in one of the pelvic bones, or "ilium" (as they are properly called); that rotation will cause you to carry your upper body weight incorrectly through your knee, thereby creating pressure and pain through your medial knee. Your medial knee will then translate that stress to the lower joints of the ankles and feet. Sometimes it occurs the other way. Unsupportive shoes, such as the ever popular flip-flops, can contribute to a dropping of the arch in the foot. If the arch is dropping, it creates a lot of pressure through the knee, which will cause the pelvis to be unstable and out of balance. An unstable pelvis will translate changes throughout the spine, up to the very first cervical vertebrae (neck bone) and can often effect your jaw. So as you can see, it's important to look at the dynamics of the entire musculoskeletal system.

Please note that I am simplifying these examples; many things can alter your biomechanics. Just for fun, begin observing people's knees; are they straight or do they bow inward or outward? Look at other's shoulders; are they even or is one higher than the other? Now, which way is the head tilted to compensate for that shoulder tilt? Consider that certain people will carry their body weight through these bowed and twisted joints for years before they feel any pain. It's no wonder that we are a society that believes vitamin A is spelled A-D-V-I-L.

To maintain healthy joints and correct biomechanical function throughout your life, you must first make certain that your skeleton is in proper alignment. Second, you will need to have toned muscles to support your skeletal system. Next, make sure that you maintain a full range of motion in all of your joint spaces. We will address the importance of exercise in the next chapter, but first you have to get your body prepared for exercise.

Exercising on a misaligned skeleton will only further degenerate your joints and supportive tissue. In order to have a full range of motion, any exercise program must take into consideration proper alignment, strength and flexibility, which will give you the ability to move freely, openly and upright. If any of these areas are a problem for you, please find a chiropractor who specializes in restoring normal motion to the joints of your body. And yes, chiropractors will adjust knees and wrists, as well as your neck and back. Ideally, when the chiropractor works on you, he will make very specific, light force adjustments. The ideal chiropractor will be a combination of a philosopher who understands that removing interference allows and helps the body to heal itself, a scientist who understands proper joint dynamics and structure, and an artist who applies a specific spinal correction to enhance your health via your nervous system—including your ability to move ... because, after all, life is motion!

Chapter 6

EXERCISE: THE ELIXIR
OF YOUTHFUL VITALITY

*I*f the fountain of youth did exist, exercise would be the water flowing through that fountain—it is that essential to good health. Exercising just 30 minutes a day, three times a week can enhance and even totally change your life for the better, starting with your energy, stamina and emotional wellbeing. In fact, a Duke University research team studied three groups of patients suffering from depression: an "exercise only" group, an "exercise plus drug therapy" group and a "drug only" group. (The antidepressant drug Zoloft was used in this study.) They found that 30 minutes of brisk exercise three times a week is just as effective as drug therapy in relieving the symptoms of major depression in the short term; however, when these people were followed for six months, only eight percent of the patients in the "exercise only" group had their depression return, while 38 percent of the "drug only" group and 31 percent of the "exercise plus drug" group relapsed.

The number one complaint that I hear from my patients (aside from "I'm in pain") is "I have no energy." With a little bit of dedication to an exercise program, your energy level can soar, and I promise that you will be thrilled with the results.

One of the greatest benefits of exercise is the ability to stave off muscle loss as we age. As mentioned in the Biomarker #1, Body cell Mass & Muscle Mass, information (see appendix) we lose an average of 6.2 pounds of muscle every decade, according to studies conducted at Tufts University's Human Nutrition and Research Center. This rate of muscle loss accelerates even more after age 45, and the only way to slow down (and even reverse) muscle loss is through purposeful muscle building exercise. Have you been actively engaged in exercise that stimulates muscle growth? If not, then this average muscle loss probably applies to you.

Please review Biomarkers 1 and 2 in the Appendix to understand how and why muscles age.

If you have been out of high school for three decades and you weigh the same as you did back then, based on averages you have probably lost approximately 18.6 pounds of muscle and replaced it with 18.6 pound of fat tissue (6.2 pounds of lost muscle mass x 3 decades = 18.6 pounds of body fat where you used to have 18.6 pounds of muscle). This creates the disease of aging called sarcopenia. Unfortunately, most of us weigh more than we did in high school, so add whatever weight you have gained since then to the 18.6 pounds of fat, and that is how much extra fat you are now carrying. Bummer, I know—but you can change it!

The Benefits of Exercise

When you consider the multitude of benefits that exercise provides, it almost seems like a miracle perscription ... and, in a way, it is. You will become biologically younger because exercise will:

- Increase your basal metabolic rate
- Increase your strength and endurance
- Increase your lean muscle mass while decreasing your body fat percentage
- Redistribute your body fat composition and improve your body shape
- Improve your insulin sensitivity
- Lower your cholesterol levels
- Reduce stress

- Increase bone density
- Improve your quality of sleep
- Increase your internal energy and vitality
- Elevate your mood naturally and more safely than artificial mood elevators
- Improve mental sharpness and concentration
- Improve your aerobic capacity
- Help normalize your blood pressure
- Improve your resting heart rate
- Help normalize your internal temperature rate (As the cardiovascular system improves through exercise, it supports temperature regulation by transferring heat produced from the muscles to the skin during exercise.)

Truthfully, if there were a pill that could do all of this, it would be malpractice not to prescribe it. Take a glance at the above list again. Every biomarker of aging is affected in a good way, as well as mood stabilization and improved mental acuity, sleep and overall energy. It's quite remarkable.

Well, exercise doesn't come in a pill form, but it is something you can manage to do by yourself and costs nothing more than a 30-minute investment of your time. Like your financial portfolio, you can always choose to invest more to experience an even greater return on your investment. Remember, your life is the sum of your choices, so as you incorporate this Biological Rejuvenation Program into your daily routine, you will want to continue to upgrade the type of exercise and increase the amount of exercise you are doing to keep your body challenged. As part of your commitment to better health, I will ask you to exercise three days every week (you can do more), concentrating on three types of activity in whatever combination you choose to do them: flexibility (stretching, range-of-motion) exercises, strengthening (resistance) exercises, and cardiovascular (aerobic) exercise.

Aerobic, Weight Resistance and Functional Training Exercise

What kind of exercise is optimal? First, it should be *aerobic*. It can be as simple as going for a daily walk by yourself or with a loved one. As you get stronger, focus on picking up the pace; look for uphill grades and begin a walk-run pattern.

Next, it is important to incorporate some type of *weight resistance* training. This is vital to maintaining or reclaiming healthy, strong bones and will help ward off osteopenia and, ultimately, osteoporosis. If you are unfamiliar with weight resistance exercise, visit <drkathleenhartford. com> for some easy-to-do home workout tips.

Functional training is an exciting classification of exercise that involves training the body for activities performed in daily life. (I suggest that you engage a chiropractor, physical therapist or personal trainer if you have not exercised in years.) Functional training can do several things for you, such as:

- Prepare you to begin an exercise program if you have not exercised for years
- Help you to rehabilitate an injured area so that you can return to the exercise or activity you love
- Prepare you for seasonal activities such as shoveling snow, starting a lawn mower and raking leaves
- Fine-tune your muscles for faster response, and increase reflexes and muscle memory
- Act as a major mojo builder!

I use this form of training to create a strong core for my patients so that they can hold their spinal corrections and create improved posture as they regain an active life. This type of exercise is also useful if your job requires you to lift heavy objects; we can target those muscles specifically. For example, if you are a hairdresser and your arms and shoulders are chronically contracted, we can target those muscles. If you love tennis but can no longer play because of shoulder pain, we will first align the shoulder and balance the muscles, then incorporate targeted exercises to strengthen the shoulder muscles. Afterwards, when you play tennis, you will be much less prone to injury—and you will enjoy having a much stronger game.

As previously mentioned, when a patient has knee pain, I align the skeleton, balance the muscles then work the muscles surrounding the knee. It seems like magic to most people; after just a few weeks of targeted functional exercise, they suddenly have no pain and can do things they haven't done in years.

We also do pre-surgical preparation—when a patient requires knee replacement surgery, for example— we work the supportive muscles of the knee joint so that they are in top shape to prepare for the changes that are about to take place. (By the way, it's important to work both knees, not just the one you are preparing for surgery.) It would be interesting to do a study of patients who've prepared for any type of surgery by getting the body to its highest level of preparatory readiness biochemically, emotionally and fitness-wise—then chart the outcomes. My guess is that the results would show a significant decrease in post-surgical infections and an accelerated recuperation. (Can you say "lowered healthcare expense"?)

The benefits of exercise can be had at any age. Rena entered my office at the age of 73 with hypothyroidism, high blood sugar, depression, hair loss, high cholesterol, no energy and a desire to lose at least 20 pounds. After 12 weeks on the Fit, Fun and Fabulous program, Rena's biological age dropped from 71 to 58. Her blood pressure lowered from 150 over 90 to 130 over 75! Rena's grip strength increased by five kilograms and she was able to perform 25 pushups instead of just three. Now, how many 73-year-olds do you know who can do that? Way to go, Rena!

Find a Form of Exercise That You Enjoy

If life is motion then exercise is "purposeful motion" that will provide all of the enormous benefits listed at the beginning of this chapter. There are many different types of exercise, and the key to staying committed is to find type or types that you enjoy. I personally enjoy dancing to upbeat music. I am also a weightlifter from way back, and I still "pump iron." My personal workout looks like this:

I divide my body into two groups, which I work with weights three to four times per week.

- Chest, legs and triceps
- Back, shoulders and biceps
- Abdominals are worked at each workout

I super-set, or do continuous sets, alternating exercises for these specific muscle groups to keep my aerobic fitness high. In other words, if I am working my chest with flies and my legs with lunges, I will move from one exercise to the next with little or no rest in between. Oftentimes, I dance from one set to another, this also supports the cardio aspect of the workout. (Well, that is the outcome, but I really do it because I like to dance! Yes, it would be embarrassing if my gym were not in my barn.)

I recently discovered that this workout just wasn't giving me the same results as it used to, even though I was changing my exercises regularly, so I incorporated a 60-second, full-out sprint on the spinning bike in between sets. This seems to be working as it keeps my energy high; it will take a few months and a few bio-impedence checks to see if I am more efficiently burning fat. Unfortunately, I had not been utilizing my fast twitch fibers (for more information on muscle fibers, see Biomarker 2) enough in my workouts over the winter months, and when I initially went to sprint, I knew it because I could feel it! So I had to target this area of endurance. My friends have been begging me to begin yoga. Although I believe it would be very beneficial, it has just never been my thing but I do enjoy pilates.

In the gym I enjoy free weights, loud music and sprints, even though I am as quiet and peaceful as a church mouse when I am not exercising. Once I am out of the gym I love hiking, off road cycling and my horse. Your exercise regime and intensity are always going to be relative to age, conditioning and the activities that you enjoy: If you are a skier, you will need to prepare for skiing; If you are a golfer, prepare for golfing; If you are a climber, prepare for climbing. Overall workouts are important, but if you want to perform well in certain activities, then prepare for them.

Possibly those most at risk for injuries are ex-athletes. Let's face it, we don't necessarily feel older in our minds, and once we begin to exercise, we start to feel much better so quickly that we may fail to allow our muscles to catch up with our minds. Shortly after you begin an exercise program, you will start to feel young again. A well-planned, systematic approach that reintroduces your body to exercise will prevent you from overdoing it and getting injured. If you are just beginning an exercise program, go to <drkathleenhartford.com> and review the exercise videos. If you are an ex-athlete, purchase a book such as *Ready, Set, Go!* by Phil Campbell and follow a program that allows you to reclaim your fitness slowly, successfully and, most importantly, without injury.

Perhaps the best plan of all would be to find a qualified personal trainer to coach you through your workouts. If you can afford it, hire a personal trainer to assist you and keep you challenged so that your body is constantly improving. Using a personal trainer even twice a month can keep your exercise program fresh and rewarding. In my office, we utilize a personal trainer to strengthen patients as they are reclaiming their biomechanical health, and I recommend that they use the trainer for exercises that will keep them moving and active at home. I suggest the same for you. It's an investment that will return to you a hundredfold in the form of good health.

Chapter 7

STRESS AND ITS EFFECTS

There is no doubt about it ... stress affects us emotionally, chemically and bio-energetically. If you really think about it—and no pun intended here—you probably couldn't come up with a time during your waking hours when your mind is at rest. It is estimated that roughly 60,000 thoughts pass through the human mind every day. Is it possible to "think" without creating a visceral (body/physical) reaction to those thoughts? Is it possible to have a visceral reaction without a bio-chemical (hormone/ neurotransmitter) response in the body? The answer to both of these questions is no—unless, perhaps, you are adept at meditation and have learned to silence your mind.

As soon as we think a thought, our body responds to it. Good thoughts release "feel good" bio-chemicals in the body; bad thoughts release "feel bad" bio-chemicals. I'm simplifying here, but it really is that simple. Our thoughts—or, more accurately, our mental/emotional interpretation of our experiences—set the stage for everything else in our lives. A person who is practiced at meditation can more readily detach from thoughts and, therefore, has little or no reaction to them—at least most of the time. (This is precisely why meditation is so valuable.) As for the rest of us, we worry, fret and obsess—and, sometimes, rightfully so. Life can be incredibly stressful, especially when things aren't going the way we think (there's that word again!) they should go.

Different Types of Stressors

Emotional Stressors

There is no doubt that life can throw us major emotional stressors, and some can be downright devastating: the death of a loved one, the loss of a job or necessary income, a child who is struggling in school or abusing substances, the loss of a home due to fire or bankruptcy, a serious accident or other health crisis. Any of these events would have a distressing effect on most of us. Hopefully, though, we learn to deal with and work through these obvious stressors and, at some point, come to peace with them.

We also carry emotional stressors brought on by our belief systems, which were probably created long before we even had a conscious understanding of them (visit <ramblingsofamadwoman.com> for more insights into this). I often say that we are trained into being; in other words, we watched how Mom and Dad handled their daily stress for about 18 years, and we've seen how relatives, teachers and friends handle their stress. Very often, we use the experiences of these people as models to help us manage our own stress ... then wake up one day saying, "Oh my God, I've become my mother / my father / my biggest fear!"

The truth of the matter is that you are not these personas or roles that you've inadvertently taken on. They are not who you really are at your core. As you become consciously aware of this, you can then chose to react differently in stressful situations. Stressors based on individual belief systems are, unfortunately, more difficult to work through, because they impact us daily in so many ways, both large and small: the irritating things our bosses or spouses do, our children's messy rooms, the traffic we deal with while commuting to work (which is always worse when we are running late!).

Daily emotional stressors are subjective depending upon each person's perception of reality, so they tend to occur again and again. For example, one person will find rush hour traffic maddening while another person enjoys it as peaceful alone time in the car, an opportunity to listen to music or books on CD that she may never have time to do otherwise. Or, you may find that Aunt Mary's nosing into your life drives you crazy, while your brother thinks she is charming, funny and means well. You may have a friend who hates balancing his checkbook but you find it to be a rewarding experience that gives you a sense of confidence and control over your finances. You see, these daily emotional stressors are based more on our perception of a situation and not necessarily a true picture of what is actually taking place. It is simply how we feel about things that are happening in our life; traffic isn't good or bad, Aunt Mary isn't good or bad, balancing your checkbook is neither good nor bad. They are what we think they are. Can we shift our perception of them? Yes, and becoming aware of a behavior pattern is the best place to start; simply allow for the possibility of perceiving things differently. Usually, this takes some time, but is well worth the effort. If this is a struggle for you, consider working with a coach or therapist. Stressors rooted in belief systems that don't serve you in living your best life can be unnecessary energy drains and, over time, can rob you of joy.

Physical Stressors

Life also brings with it physical stress. The body does its best to respond to physical stressors with healthy adaptive responses, but if they continue unchecked for a long period of time, they can and will wear your body down. For instance, the body adapts to the stress of cold temperature by creating goose bumps or shivering; hot temperatures produce sweating; viral stressors such as the seasonal flu cause a healthy body to create antibodies and a fever to kill the virus (yes, the fever is there for a reason). Even some forms of exercise, such as lifting weights, stress our muscles; in response, the body will create new muscle tissue so that it can handle the weight the next time it has to experience it. A healthy body will adapt to physical stressors provided that it has the support it needs in the form of nutrients and rest, and provided that the stress does not continue for a prolonged period of time. That is, if you cannot get warm in a freezing cold environment, you will experience hypothermia. If you lift weight too hard and too long and do not provide the body with the necessary repair nutrients for the muscles or the necessary rest for repair, the muscles will begin to break down. If you are exposed to a virus and do not support the immune system in its effort to eradicate the virus, the body will become sick. Have you noticed that not everybody who is exposed to a virus gets the virus? As human beings, we have limitations as to what our bodies can endure physically, spiritually and emotionally. If left unsupported for the long term, these stressors will slowly wear the body, and out spirit, down.

This is what happened with my patient Jen, who was only 36 years old when she came to my office. She was experiencing neck, shoulder and lower back discomfort, digestive bloating and irregularity, and her biological age came in at 51. As we spoke, what came to light was that the stress in Jen's life was off the charts; in fact, she was having recurring nightmares from it all. Even though Jen was not overweight, she understood that health is a balance of all systems, so she committed to the Fit, Fun and Fabulous program. By the end of the 12 weeks, all of her chief complaints had subsided and her biological and chronological ages aligned. Essentially, Jen had recovered 15 years of biological youth and was able to handle the stressors in her life much better.

Metabolic Stressors

Other types of stressors can affect the body in similar, yet often unknown, ways. Metabolic stressors are things such as free radicals, nutrient deficiencies, pharmaceutical medications, poor diet and toxins in the environment. Traditional medicine can be very limited in its treatment and management of the above stressors; in fact, sometimes the medical community's approach might even create and contribute to these stressors by adding additional drugs to a person's already struggling system. Remember, medicine is the diagnosis and treatment of disease, and sometimes physicians have to utilize aggressive procedures and powerfully toxic pharmaceuticals to achieve that goal. This is why it is very beneficial to have a natural integrative healthcare professional on your team. There may be times when you need medical intervention, and an integrative practitioner can help you prepare for a planned surgical or invasive procedure. Once the procedure is complete, the integrative practitioner can help support your healing process so that you can return to a fully active life with the least possible side effects.

We mentioned earlier about the desirability of preoperative preparation for an orthopedic surgical procedure, say a hip or knee replacement. There are several things that you would want to do. First, as much as possible, strengthen the muscles around the joint that will be replaced and provide nutrients to support this strengthening; second, support the gut (intestinal tract) with targeted nutrients, such as anti-inflammatory medical foods, and probiotics, to offset the antibiotics that you will require during the surgical procedure and the inflammation created any type an invasive or traumatic event occurs in the body. While you are in the hospital, I suggest that all natural therapies be stopped because they tend to confuse the physicians, and it is best at this time to let them do their thing ... but you, the patient, should know what that thing is. In a perfect world, your traditional physician and your natural integrative physician would communicate on all levels of your care—but until they do, it is your responsibility to know what is being done to your body so that your natural integrative physician can help to offset the side effects of necessary medications. Any medical procedure being performed should have a pre- and post-procedure natural approach to aid the body in cleansing, healing and repairing tissue.

Bio-energetic Stressors

Bio-energetic stressors are another important consideration. We all have an energetic thumbprint, which can be interfered with by things like fluorescent lights, computers, cell phones and cell phone towers. To understand this, let's first define what electric and magnetic fields actually are. Electricity is the movement of electrons, or current, through a wire. The type of electricity that runs through power lines and houses is alternating current (AC). AC power produces two types of fields, or "areas of energy"—an electric field and a magnetic field. These two fields together are referred to as electric and magnetic fields, or EMFs. Both electric and magnetic fields are present around appliances and power lines. Electric fields are easily shielded or weakened by walls and other objects; magnetic fields, on the other hand, can pass through buildings, human bodies and most other materials. Since magnetic fields are most likely to penetrate the body, they are the component of EMFs that are usually studied in relation to cancer.

The focus of most research studies related to EMFs and cancer has been on extremely low-frequency magnetic fields, such as power lines and electrical appliances like shavers, hair dryers, computers, televisions, electric blankets and heated waterbeds—and whether these fields can cause childhood cancers, especially brain tumors and leukemia. I am sure you have also heard conflicting reports about cell phone usage and its possible connection to brain tumors. This field of study is very new, much like the bio-energetic healing approaches that I feel will be the medicine of the future. I would like to suggest that perhaps the problem lies not just with cell phones or electrical wires, but rather with the toxic load that is created by the combination of multiple factors. Coupled with poor food choices, powerful medications, environmental toxins, and genetic or created weaknesses in the body, it is this toxic load that creates many of our health issues. What can be done about this? While there is no one cause or cure for these toxic loads, a continuous attempt to manage them through programs like *Fit, Fun and Fabulous* can be highly beneficial.

Feel Your Feelings!

I spoke a few pages ago about stressors formed from our own belief systems. Yes, any kind of emotional charge will affect you energetically. These stressful thoughts can change your energetic thumbprint and release hormones and other biochemicals. Whether it's feeling brokenhearted or getting a gut instinct about something, these feelings are real to you and your body. Do not ignore your feelings! Your body does not lie, and it has a way of knowing things on a molecular level, oftentimes before we are able to consciously tap into it. If you have discomfort in a certain area, feel congested or your body feels restricted in some way, pay attention to the subtle signs that your body is giving you.

All stressors create a fight-or-flight primal response in the body. This is healthy and provides the extra energy needed to handle any imminent threat. It makes us feel alive and powerful and energetic. Unfortunately, many of us get addicted to this extra boost of adrenaline from our workouts, our emotional upsets or our work, and we create an imbalance by wanting more of that "high." We over-train, overwork or argue about everything. It becomes particularly destructive in personal relationships when repeated drama is created. Our conversations tend to center around what is wrong in our lives instead of what is right and good.

Eventually, this leads to burnout, insulin resistance and oftentimes an anti-climactic feeling that can closely resemble depression. The stress response releases hormones that can affect bodily functions such as digestion, relaxation and cellular repair. The involuntary fight-or-flight response is there to protect you against emergency situations for survival, such as a grizzly bear in the woods—not against an ongoing conflict with a spouse, co-worker or family member. When we live in a heightened adrenaline state, the chronic adrenal stress depletes our body's reserves and accelerates the aging process. Unresolved emotional drama and conflicts can make you old before your time! So how do we combat stress? Let's take a look at that now.

Stress Management

It's amusing how life sometimes works. As I was preparing to write this section, I had a string of extremely stressful days. Perhaps I was being given a chance to practice what I'm about to share.

As previously pointed out, our fast-paced modern world tends to turn most areas of our lives into a fight-or-flight situation. This innate response helps us to handle life-threatening events, but it does nothing to help the body digest food, get proper sleep or repair cells. Several things happen when we are in the fight-or-flight mode. The sympathetic nervous system becomes dominant; first, blood is sent to the extremities so that the muscles in the arms and legs will be ready and able to fight a threat or flee from danger. The pupils dilate to broaden the eyes' range of vision and focus. The torso twists so that if we fight or are attacked, vital organs will be protected from a direct blow. We clench our jaw to protect our head and tighten the shoulders so that we can raise our arms in self-defense or strike a blow to our opponent—much like a boxer's stance. All of this helps us to survive while under attack.

The body perceives emotional attacks, work deadlines and other varieties of stress in much the same way. It's no wonder that we (and our children) have digestive and sleep disorders, neck tension and headaches, and feel exhausted and depressed. We gain weight and even subconsciously grind our teeth while supposedly at rest. It's a direct result of today's lifestyle. We are constantly on the run and driving in our cars. We seldom sit down for a quiet, healthy meal. How can we with deadlines to meet and to-do lists to accomplish? For goodness' sake, we carry our office in our phone, constantly receiving emails, texts and voice messages that set us up to add more tasks to our to-do lists. We run our children from activity to activity while they text friends and manage their social network from their phones. We model to them that this hyper-manic state of "doingness" is normal ... and it never ends. In such a cortisol-induced state, the body struggles to de-stress, digest food, heal, repair and detoxify so that it can do the one thing it is made to do: survive!

Cortisol is a hormone that the body releases in response to stress. It counteracts insulin, greatly contributing to your cells' insulin-resistance which, in turn, contributes to hyperglycemia (high blood sugar). It also acts as a diuretic that suppresses the immune system by inhibiting T-cell production; it reduces calcium absorption and even interferes with the reproductive system. As you can imagine, inappropriate levels of cortisol play a major role in accelerating the aging process. So naturally, part of stress management is managing our cortisol (we will explore this in Chapter 8).

Shift Your Perspective

To begin to manage stress, we have to be realistic about how we perceive the world. Until we can shift our perspective—which can only be done through continuous awareness and internal/personal growth work—Aunt Mary is going to drive you crazy, your boss is going to be a demanding and aggressive SOB, and your children will continue to push your buttons. Add this stress, on top of feminine hormone changes or major life events, and you have a formula for daily drama and frustration.

Of course, stress affects the mind as well as the body. Continuous stress can create mental confusion. Often what you think you are upset about has nothing to do with what you say it is. For instance, that demanding boss frustrates and angers you every day at work, but he is your boss and there is nothing you can say. So every night, Monday through Friday, you go home emotionally upset, and the first person you see is your spouse. Then the weekend arrives. You come home from grocery shopping and greet your spouse. Suddenly you feel … that's right … angry and frustrated! Your poor hubby or wife has done nothing to activate these feelings, but he or she has been the first person you saw at the end of each very difficult and irritating work day. At some point, then, just seeing his or her face will trigger these feelings within you, and you begin to believe that your spouse is the cause of your inner turmoil. Before you know it—bingo!—you have created marital problems that really have nothing to do with your marriage!

Our lives are a continuous and complex series of stimulation and response—a roller coaster of emotions. Throughout these chapters, I offer proven techniques and approaches that will have profoundly positive results on your stress levels. I hope that it is now clear to you that stress occurs when: (1) the body is compromised through nerve system interference, biochemical stressors (from food, medications and the environment), as well as emotional stressors from our daily demands and perceptions of life; and (2) the body does not receive the necessary support to offset these stressors.

Manage Stress with 10 Lifestyle Habits of Biological Rejuvenation

Now, let's review the *Fit, Fun and Fabulous* lifestyle's 10 habits of biological rejuvenation.

1. Balanced eating
2. Eating frequency
3. Regular exercise
4. Reduced stimulant use
5. Stress management
6. Supplement balance

7. Hormone balance
8. Musculoskeletal balance
9. Quality sleep
10. Hydration

All of these health enhancers support the rejuvenation process at the cellular level, and when combined they will help you to manage stress.

Balanced eating and eating frequency are the top 2 of the list for a reason; they are your foundation! By following the food guidelines listed in this Biological Rejuvenation Program, you will support your body's ability to handle stress. With the proper nutrients, you will experience less dramatic increases in stress-related hormones—particularly cortisol which, as mentioned, contributes greatly to accelerated aging. You will also avoid the heightened hypoglycemic response of simple carbohydrate food and the inevitable sluggishness, mind fog and fatigue caused by their metabolism.

Exercise is number three on the list for a reason; it is vital because life is motion! In addition to helping with biological rejuvenation, exercise is a great stress reliever and blood sugar modulator. Studies show that even a 10-minute brisk walk—perhaps at lunchtime, first thing in the morning or right after work—will do wonders for lowering your stress level. Even if you think that your schedule does not allow for the recommended exercise of 30 to 40 minutes a day, you can surely find five or 10 minutes to do a simple power walk, jog in place or do a set of jumping jacks, like in gym class. If you commit to even 10-minute segments of exercise, your body will soon feel the benefits of increased energy and well being, as you release a host of 'feel good' endorphins and you will begin to crave more of that feeling. Once you enjoy the positive experience of exercise in your daily routine, it will become easier to find ways to create more time to commit to it.

Sleep is perhaps the most important stress reliever and health enhancer, and it's something that we can enjoy at no risk and no cost. Remember, we have two nervous systems that must maintain balance: the sympathetic nervous system and the parasympathetic nervous system. Fight-or-flight is a response from the sympathetic nervous system. In the parasympathetic nervous system, the opposite happens. The body becomes quiet and the heart rate slows down to prepare the body to relax, heal and repair itself. Blood is directed to your core to aid in digestion and move nutrients throughout the body for cellular repair and detoxification. The body is meant to activate the parasympathetic nervous system after meals; this is why many countries still have siesta time and why power naps are so rejuvenating. This is also why high-powered business lunches usually cause indigestion, which can lead to ulcers over long periods of time.

The work of the parasympathetic nervous system is most pronounced during the night when the body is at rest. Oftentimes, working late at night will interfere with sleep, which adds to our stress level. Some companies, such as Google, are supporting this concept with "sleep pods" where employees can enjoy power naps. Studies show that 20 minutes of sleep in the afternoon provides more rest than an additional 20 minutes of sleep in the morning (although the last two hours of morning sleep have special benefits of their own). The body seems to be designed for this, as most people naturally become tired in the afternoon, about eight hours after waking up.

Other things that can interfere with sleep include the following:

- Irregular sleep patterns, especially shift work or changing your sleep times. Try to maintain a consistent sleep schedule.
- Intensive physical or mental activity within three or four hours of bedtime.
- Consumption of caffeine or alcohol several hours prior to bedtime. Consider drinking a relaxing herbal tea instead.
- Heavy meals prior to bedtime. If possible, eat a light meal of protein and vegetables by 7 p.m. and avoid late night snacking.
- Especially for ladies: Chinese medicine has demonstrated that the liver meridian can be stressed during times of hormonal fluctuations, Ovulation, PMS, Menopause creating night time insomnia between the hours of 1 and 3 a.m.

Meditation and Simple Relaxation Techniques

Simple relaxation techniques also help to manage stress. I cannot say enough about the benefits of meditation. Some people are uncomfortable with this term, perhaps Mother Theresa's explanation will put your mind at ease, "Prayer is when I talk to God; meditation is when I listen." We have so many tentacles attached to our children, our spouses, our jobs, our challenges and upsets. Of course, we need to be involved in many of these areas but, for just 20 minutes a day, if we can draw that energy back to our heart center and simply feel in tune with ourselves and our dreams, we can create a completely different day and, ultimately, a completely different life. Try it. It is so powerful to tune in each day to a higher power that lives inside of you, to experience the oneness and stillness of life before becoming engaged in the world. Doing so is mentally, physically and spiritually profound.

We also need to look at the relationships we have with others and ourselves. Surround yourself with supportive, life-enhancing people. If you repeatedly feel exhausted after interacting with a friend or colleague, you're probably better off distancing yourself from that person. If you feel completely drained by your thoughts, then change them. Again, meditation can help you clear your mind, shift behavior patterns and make better choices about relationships and inner fears.

If meditation is challenging for you, try journaling. This is another effective, low-cost activity for managing stress. The act of writing down your thoughts moves the energy from inside of your body to the outside; this helps to provide a different perspective on whatever topic you're journaling about. Journaling will help to bring a new idea, dream or desire into the physical world in the form of words. If you are working through an emotionally upsetting issue, journaling can help you process your feelings, helping to alleviate stressful thoughts and bringing a measure of peace to both mind and body. Journaling is also a wonderful tool to review your day, release all thoughts and drop into a deep, relaxing sleep. I believe so strongly in journaling that I created a *Fit, Fun and Fabulous Journal* to coincide with this book. This journal allows you to follow your food intake, thought patterns, exercise activities and rest time. Your journal will give you the opportunity to celebrate your day and all that you have accomplished. (This journal can be ordered at <drkathleenhartford.com>.)

Bodywork

The many types of bodywork available today can help manage stress, as well.

As mentioned in Chapter 5, *chiropractic* care is a very effective way to manage and control the physical manifestations of emotional and physical stress. Chiropractic balances the sympathetic and parasympathetic nervous system response while releasing muscle fatigue and spasm.

Massage is another excellent stress reducer. It supports balanced muscles along with blood and lymphatic flow; it also feels really good and allows you to rest for at least 30 minutes.

A type of bodywork called *biofeedback* gives you greater control over your physical responses to mental and emotional stimuli. It teaches you how to identify and control your inside world through listening to your body's biological feedback and managing its responses.

A wonderful technique called *neuro-emotional technique* can help you uncover the originating events that have created certain ways of being in your life. This technique can not only balance the energy behind the event but also break the neurological loop that keeps the mind's tape running, causing us to continue to repeatedly think the same thoughts and react in the same ways.

Dr Darren Weissman's *Life Line Technique* is another cutting edge approach to transform the health of your body and your relationships. (visit our podcasts to listen to a conversation with Dr. Weismann on my Health Pyramid Radio Show <www.drkathleenhartford.com>

Tell the Truth

Here is another suggestion for releasing stress in your life: learn to tell the truth. You know, so often we try to spare someone's feelings by telling little white lies. It sounds something like this: "No, really, it's okay" or "Sure, I have time to help you again." To avoid conflict, we lie. Although seemingly innocent or noble, these little mistruths can accumulate and create resentment in your relationships, as well as exhaustion in yourself. When you take on more responsibility than you should, you inevitably hit a breaking point and risk doing irreparable damage to the relationship.

Just tell the truth, which would sound something like this: "No, I'm sorry, I really can't" or "Honey, I love you but when you do that I feel like ... " (fill in the blank). No shouting or drama is necessary; a simple "yes," "no," "please" or "thank you" will set you free. Just try it. I promise, you *will* live through it and will have a more authentic life for it.

Time Management

Learning how to manage your time effectively can be a great stress reducer. So much of our stress comes from being overwhelmed with projects, appointments and various commitments. Get real with yourself. Buy a calendar; in fact, your phone probably has one. Chart out the real time required to perform tasks and plan your days. There is an old saying in the scuba diving community: Plan your dive and dive your plan. In other words, stick to it. Have boundaries. Don't get distracted or you will get in trouble. Be honest with yourself as to what you can and cannot do, and let others adapt to that. It is not your job to make their lives work for them, but it is your job to keep your word—so don't say you will do something if you can't. If you've promised to do it, then do your best—but learn to ask for help, if needed.

Leisure Activities

Finally, develop hobbies and leisurely activities, and support your loved ones in doing the same—even if their interests don't include you. Gardening, golfing, hiking and weekend trips all break up patterns of constant stimulation and allow you to relax and return to your life refreshed and renewed. Living a *Fit, Fun and Fabulous* life as the best most authentic YOU will be a reward all its own!

Chapter 8

HORMONE BALANCING

ormone balancing is an important yet complex topic, because it encompasses a complete study of medicine called endocrinology. Volumes could be written about this subject, but for the purpose of incorporating this Biological Rejuvenation Program into your life, I will focus here on the basic function of the hormones: insulin, cortisol, glucagon, estrogen and xenoestrogens.

Insulin

I cannot emphasize enough the importance of balanced *insulin*. Allow me to take a minute to explore with you some very common areas where we get in trouble with our choices. Let's say you begin or end your day feeling a little tired or a bit blue. You know that piece of chocolate or doughnut is going to make you feel better. And you know what? It does. Carbohydrate-loading of high-glycemic food can trigger a blood sugar spike, which creates a short-lived energy boost and releases a "feel good" neurotransmitter called serotonin. Serotonin acts as a mood enhancer for the short period of time that it's present in your system—about 20 minutes. After 20 minutes of feeling good, your blood sugar will begin to plummet as your body pumps insulin to the blood to reduce the sugar released by these simple carbohydrates. When your blood sugar begins to drop, you start to feel lethargic, even mildly depressed. In order to feel good once again, you reach for another cookie, more potato chips or other carbohydrates to regain that temporary high and false sense of energy. In about another 20 minutes, you're back to square one ... and as with most addictions, it leaves you feeling empty and wanting more again and again.

This insulin imbalance is one very important cause of the carbohydrate cravings that so many people struggle with; in fact, those who have eaten a high carbohydrate meal will eat on average 200 more calories in their next meal than someone following a low carbohydrate/low glycemic meal plan. As you can imagine, this carb roller coaster eventually leads to unwanted weight gain, because when insulin levels are high you deposit more fat, and when blood sugar levels plummet you feel lethargic and melancholy—not a good mood to be in when you need to get up and exercise or simply be active.

Because of this continuous cycle of simple carbohydrate consumption, the body begins to require more insulin than is healthy in order to handle these higher-than-normal blood sugar levels; this results in insulin resistance. When this occurs long term, the pancreas burns out and you become Type 2 diabetic. What's more, this insulin damages the arterial walls and in order to protect these walls, the body releases a sticky substance called cholesterol. Cholesterol serves as an adhesive bandage to repair the arterial wall. As this bandaging effect creates rigidity in the arterial walls, the blood pressure begins to rise. High insulin levels also affect blood pressure in another way. It prevents the storage of magnesium and, as a result, this magnesium passes out of the body through urination. Magnesium stored in your cells relaxes your muscles. If your magnesium level is too low, your blood vessels will constrict rather than relax, which will raise your blood pressure, decrease your energy level and cause an imbalance with calcium. Low levels of magnesium will also leave you constipated and depressed. Insulin also affects your blood pressure by causing your body to retain sodium. Sodium retention causes fluid retention. Fluid retention, in turn, causes high blood pressure and can ultimately lead to congestive heart failure. Thus begins the downward spiral of metabolic syndrome and accelerated aging.

Cortisol

We have already touched on cortisol, the hormone that the body releases in response to stress. Cortisol is a corticosteroid hormone that is produced by the adrenal cortex. It is elevated in the morning to help you start your day and should decline by nightfall. Studies show that it is more elevated in women than men, especially working women. This may be due to the fact that many women come home from work and dive right into household and family duties. Women also tend to multi-task, not only in their activities but also in their heads.

It is almost impossible to avoid stress. Finding ways to mitigate it in our lives, however, is important. As we've already discussed, stress can create havoc on our health in so many ways. For example, the more chronic our stress becomes, the more fat we accumulate around the mid-section. New studies demonstrate that elevated cortisol levels can lead not only to abdominal weight gain, but also to the loss of verbal declarative memory (words, names and numbers). Stress also creates insulin resistance and can lead to Type 2 diabetes and heart disease. Remember what was said earlier about metabolic syndrome? Cortisol is very important in relation to metabolic syndrome and the hormonal cascade that occurs during stressful times. Cortisol becomes elevated when we do not get adequate amounts of sleep, and we all know that stress oftentimes makes it more difficult to sleep. Cortisol can also play a factor in fertility, bone health, the immune system, high blood pressure and ... can you say "accelerated aging"?

Glucagon

Glucagon serves a major role in maintaining normal levels of blood sugar. As you now know, your body requires that your blood glucose level be maintained in a very specific and narrow range. This range is regulated by two hormones: insulin and glucagon. Insulin is produced by the beta cells of the pancreas in response to high blood sugar levels, while glucagon is produced by the alpha cells of the pancreas in response to low blood sugar levels. When insulin is released in response to high blood sugar levels, fat cells will take in glucose from the blood; this is how we increase our fat stores. When our blood sugar level is too low, glucagon is released and the liver is signaled to release glucose into the blood stream. We also release glucagon following a high protein meal in response to high levels of amino acids in the blood.

Glucagon can also be released in response to exercise. It is not actually clear whether the stimulus is the exercise per se or the accompanying exercise-induced depletion of glucose. As you exercise, two things happen: your blood sugar is depleted as it is used for energy, and your muscle tissue breaks down, which releases amino acids. Glucagon responds to both of these things. The good news is that those amino acids will then be used to recreate muscle tissue. This is why you must break down muscle to build muscle; bodybuilders and other high-performance athletes are effective at utilizing this process to create increased muscle mass and strength. Working the muscles creates stress on the bones, which signals the body that a new bone matrix needs to be laid down which will enable the bones to handle the additional load being placed on them. This is how targeted muscle-building exercise helps to prevent and reverse bone thinning improving our 10th biomarker Bone Mineral density.

Glucogon secretion, on the other hand, is inhibited by high levels of blood sugar, such as after eating a high-carbohydrate meal. This is another good reason to avoid high-glycemic foods. Just keep this in mind: as blood sugar increases, fat stores increase, as well.

Estrogen

Many women seem to have a love-hate relationship with this hormone. If you are bloated, emotional and waiting for your monthly cycle to start, you probably hate it. If you are menopausal and estrogen saves you from getting hot flashes, you probably love it. Unfortunately, hormone replacement therapy (HRT) and birth control pills have been shown to alter gut flora and compromise the immune system (much like antibiotics). They have also been linked to the creation of reproductive cancers within the body. These medications, like all medications, must be given very serious consideration prior to their use.

Other conditions that are related to or exacerbated by estrogen imbalance are PMS, endometriosis, uterine fibroid tumors, fibrocystic breasts and cervical dysplasia. These are issues that many women have to deal with throughout their lives. Rest assured that there are many natural approaches to balancing hormones without resorting to potential cancer-causing prescriptions for HRT or birth control. Targeted nutrients such as indole-3-carbinol, rhaportic rhubarb, rosemary and flax can support the balancing of estrogen.

Targeted nutrients for liver detoxification are equally important for supporting the conjugation of estrogen. The liver must be able to effectively conjugate our hormones and when it cannot do this effectively, it can create an estrogen-dominant state within the body. Estrogen dominant states, especially from synthetic estrogens or any estrogen that is not made naturally by the body, have been proven to cause cancer.

Xenoestrogens

Xenoestrogens are foreign estrogens in the environment that mimic the body's natural hormones. These industrially produced estrogens' ability to mimic our natural hormones creates a clogging of our receptor sites and interferes with the body's ability to utilize its natural hormones; this can lead to many types of environmental cancers. Gentlemen, this information is relevant to you, as well; these estrogen mimickers can affect the male body, leaving it vulnerable to estrogen-induced cancers and fertility issues. These hormones can be directly affected by your life choices and your environment. Working in certain industrial environments, drinking from plastic water bottles that have been reused or sitting in a warm vehicle, even microwaving food in plastic containers can release xenoestrogens into your body.

According to the American Cancer Society, environmental toxins like xenoestrogens can have an estrogenic effect on the body, whether male or female. These estrogen-like chemicals may be the cause of increased prevalence of reproductive cancers, such as breast, testicular and prostate. In fact, reproductive-related cancers have been linked to estrogen compounds since the 1970s. Recent studies have shown that sperm count is 50 percent less than it was 50 years ago, the incidence of testicular cancer has tripled, and prostate cancer has doubled during that same time. In 1960, the occurrence of breast cancer was one in 20; now it is one in eight. This is especially true in Florida where pesticide use is high. Many of the alligators have been rendered sexually unable to function because of the pesticides leaching into the waterways and affecting the growth of their reproductive organs.

I see numerous complaints in my office that may be related to xenoestrogens and their effect on our receptor sites. Xenoestrogens are very effective endocrine (hormone) disrupters because they mimic our hormones so effectively that they are able to attach to the receptor site on the cell wall, which is meant to accept only our hormones. This is how your hormones activate the cell. It is a lock and key system, but xenoestrogens can mimic that hormonal key. You see, it's the hormone's ability to attach to the cell's receptor site that will determine the activity and effectiveness of your hormones, not the level of hormones in your blood stream. If the hormones cannot connect to receptor sites, it's like they aren't even there—but if you check blood values, they may be normal. The result, ultimately, is that the ability of our own hormones to activate our cells will be compromised, and you will have all of the symptoms of someone with a glandular problem, but your blood values will be in the normal range.

Men and women with fertility issues due to endocrine disrupters are common, but perhaps the most common complaint I hear is women with suspected thyroid issues. They enter my office complaining that they have gone to their medical doctor, certain that they have a thyroid problem. They explain to the doctor, "I am always tired" ... "My hair is falling out" ... "I've put on so much weight" ... "I'm constantly freezing" ... "I have absolutely no energy" ... "I feel moderately depressed all the time" ... "I feel like my head is in a fog and I can't concentrate." The doctor may then run a thyroid panel and will probably say the thyroid is fine; then to pacify the patient, he may diagnose her with mild depression and prescribe an antidepressant. Unfortunately, this may cause additional weight gain, and weight gain usually makes the depression worse. After going through this process, the woman eventually walks into my office frustrated and hopeless, praying as a last resort that I can do something to help.

The medical doctor is correct: the thyroid, for now, is fine. It is pumping out hormones as fast as it can, but the receptor sites are not open and available for the hormones to enter and activate the cells. You cannot put another key in a lock that already has a key in it. In other words, the thyroid hormone cannot attach to the cell wall to activate the cell and provide you with the benefit of thyroid hormones if the receptor sites are filled with environmental hormone mimickers. The hormone levels in the blood do not indicate what is available to the cells. This is very important to understand. Hormone levels in the blood are oftentimes likened to people in a shopping mall parking lot during the Christmas holiday rush. They drive in circles around the lot because they can't find a spot; until they can park, walk into the mall and shop, they cannot activate their buying power. This is similar to what occurs with a cell; the blood does not show the availability of the hormone to activate the cell. When the hormone is not able to adhere to and activate the cell, your symptoms are the same as they would be if no hormone was present at all.

Women tell me all the time, "I have been going to the doctor for years and he keeps telling me that my thyroid levels are fine." If you wait long enough, your thyroid will eventually exhaust and you will become hypothyroid. Finally, the doctor will give you a prescription for thyroid hormones to go along with your antidepressant. If your problem is actually an endocrine disruptor issue, and not a hormone production issue, then your receptor sites will be no more available for the prescribed hormones than they were for your own thyroid hormones. Your blood values will improve, however, and because of that, your doctor will say that you should be feeling better. Unfortunately, you are still not able to activate the cell at the receptor site. The poor women in this situation are left feeling exhausted, unattractive from losing their hair and miserable from putting on weight almost uncontrollably—and yet they have no energy to exercise.

So what is the solution? There is help for all of these conditions: targeted nutrients along with some very effective therapeutic techniques that can change your life. We will get there but before we do, let's first look at how body shapes play into hormone balancing and much more.

Chapter 9

BODY SHAPES

As a healthcare provider, I believe it is important to take a holistic approach to patient care, similar to "back in the day" when doctors spent one-on-one time with their patients, rather than relying solely on diagnostic tests to tell them what their patients required. I also believe that the commercial programming toward 'every ill has a pill', a chronically sick, stressed and obese nation and the threat of potential law suits have greatly dehumanized the doctor-patient relationship. I had a wonderful primary care physician when I was a child; he looked at me and talked to me, and I felt he cared deeply for me. (His name was Dr. John Pacek, and I'd like to acknowledge the doctor-patient relationship he modeled for me.)

As a chiropractor, when I spend time with my patients, the first thing I notice is their gait as they walk into my office—head position and tilt, shoulder heights and foot angles. I look at how the knee is working in relation to the pelvis and foot and, of course, any restrictions in motion as the patient moves. I also look at the health of the my clients' hair, skin and nails, as these can tell me a lot about their internal health conditions. The tongue, in particular, can give an enormous amount of information about the state of one's health, as do the whites of the eyes and fingernails. When it comes to any environmental or chemical stressors or imbalances that a person might be experiencing, it is actually body shape that gives me initial clues as to what organ or system might be requiring initial attention.

Thyroid Body Type

In the last chapter, I mentioned that many people believe they have a problem with their thyroid gland even when their blood values continue to be in a normal range. A *Thyroid Body Type* does exist, and I will rely on that assessment before any blood tests for all of the reasons outlined in the previous chapter. When a person with a *Thyroid Body Type* gains weight, it is throughout the entire body—from shoulders to hips. The body takes on an upward rectangular shape that is sometimes referred to as a "fire plug" appearance. This person's gait is characterized by an arm swing in which the thumb turns inward toward the thigh. Their symptoms are typically:

- Hair loss
- Exhaustion
- Freezing on the inside, to their core
- Uncontrollable cravings for carbohydrates, especially at night
- Difficulty falling asleep at night, especially between the hours of 9 and 11pm, due to endocrine meridian imbalance
- Thought patterns that create ongoing confusion
- Difficulty focusing and completing tasks

They may also suffer from high cholesterol, decreased libido, a weak heart and loose, flabby skin. Individuals with this body type may have tried everything to lose weight, but the truth is, they are too exhausted to even think about exercise; they tend to self-sabotage by reaching for the creamy carbohydrates to sooth their lowered self-esteem.

Adrenal Body Types

The *Adrenal Body Types* are very similar to the metabolic syndrome or blood sugar destabilization body type. These individuals have been chronically in fight-or-flight mode and are now feeling burned out. When they were young, they were thin, high strung, loved stimulants and thrived on stress. These individuals burn the candle at both ends and, as they get older, the adrenal system begins to suffer under the strain. Because this body type doesn't typically experience problems with weight or energy levels earlier in life, these individuals struggle with the changes in their bodies once they get older. They are frustrated that they cannot do the things they used to do. Do you know someone who often tells stories such as, "When I was younger, I could ... stay up all night ... climb mountains and hike for hours ... clean the house from top to bottom without stopping"? This person is most probably an adrenal body type. Over time, the adrenal system begins to burn out, which results in an inability to handle stress. This leads to things like jumping at an unexpected noise, weight gain around the mid-section, fluid retention, dehydration, cellular wall resistance to nutrients and inflammatory pain. Altered pH due to the acidity caused from prolonged stress, sometimes also results in calcium deposits. These body types truly feel burned out, with little energy to do what they used to love. They usually crave salt, have trouble falling asleep, cannot turn off their thoughts, are prone to worry and tend to be hypoglycemic (low blood sugar), resulting in light-headedness with changes in posture, potential headaches and overall low energy.

Liver / Toxicity Body Types

Liver or *Toxicity Body Types* are people who have usually been around toxic environments, have ingested excessive amounts of medication, or have generally followed a very unhealthy lifestyle, oftentimes involving alcohol. This body type will have a pot belly that looks like a "swallowed basketball." The skin tends to look unhealthy. (The skin is the body's largest detoxification organ—yes, the skin is an organ—which performs a multitude of functions, not the least of which is producing vitamin D and handling the overflow of toxins in your system.) This is another reason why it is important for doctors to look at their patients. The skin, along with previously mentioned indicators, gives us a clear insight into a patient's health. We can see what is going on with a patient long before a medical test confirms that there is a problem. It is possible to see problems as they are being created. By utilizing integrated wellness care approaches, we can often address and correct problems long before they require medical intervention.

Such is the case with the *Liver Body Type*. These individuals will often:
- Wake up between 1 and 3 a.m. and have trouble falling back to sleep
- Experience joint pain, inflammation and stiffness, especially with their initial movement
- Tend toward anger and can become depressed
- Crave fatty food but usually suffer with indigestion and tend to bloat, belch and burp following their meals
- Have skin problems and are usually swollen in their appearance, in their joints and under their eyes
- Have a full feeling under their right rib cage
- In prolonged cases, have a yellow tint in the whites of their eyes

At times, body types and symptoms will overlap. An example of this would be during a time of hormonal swings. Since the liver is responsible for conjugating your hormones, during times of hormonal fluctuations such as menopause, pre-menstruation or pre-ovulation, several things may happen (which an integrative healthcare practitioner can help you address). You may tend to:
- Crave things you do not normally crave, like chocolate
- Experience breakouts on your face
- Wake up or experience insomnia between 1 and 3 a.m.
- Have hormonal headaches (on the top of your head)
- Experience the "emotions" of the liver

The emotional aspect of health is where integrative medicine gets really interesting. According to traditional Chinese medicine (TCM), the emotions associated with liver chi stagnation are anger, resentment, gall (as in, "How dare you!"), stubbornness, repressed emotions, depression, indecision, irrationality, frustration and aggression—not that any of us has ever experienced those emotions during times of heightened hormonal levels!

Reproductive Hormone Body Type

In my workshops, when I ask the audience if anyone has experienced the following list of emotions during a time of reproductive hormonal changes, the women laugh and the men shake their heads because they are afraid to laugh. The *Reproductive Hormone Body Type* will experience:

- Weight gain mostly around the lower abdominal area and upper thighs
- Feeling hormonally out of balance
- Hormonal headaches on the top of the head
- Mood swings related to monthly ovulation or menstrual cycle
- Extreme physical and emotional swings with menopause
- Chocolate cravings, especially during hormonal fluctuations
- Fluid retention, mostly in the hands

Many factors can contribute to reproductive hormonal imbalances and, make no mistake, this happens with both men and women. In fact, the BP oil spill that our country experienced in 2010 could create xenoestrogenic effects in our body, because petrochemicals are estrogenic in nature. In other words, we have environmental toxins surrounding us that will affect our estrogen levels and estrogen receptors, which will create higher-than-normal concentrations of estrogen in both men and women. (Read more about xenoestrogens in Chapter 8.)

Even FDA-approved pharmaceutical estrogen compounds can create cancer in the human body. The "Million Women Study" (actually, it was 948,576 post-menopausal women) conducted in the United Kingdom was published in *The Lancet* on April 10, 2007. In this study, half of the women took Hormone Replacement Therapy (HRT) for at least five years. The study followed these women for 5.3 years to check the rate of ovarian cancer, and 6.9 years to check for mortality. The women using HRT were 23 percent more likely to die of ovarian cancer. Bad enough, but when they added the risk of endometrial and breast cancer, the risk increased to 63 percent. Obviously, that's worse than 50:50 odds.

In fact, when it comes to cancer deaths, it is stated in the book *The Secret War on Cancer* that there have been 10 million preventable cancer deaths during the past 30 years. This huge amount of preventable deaths, if nothing else, shows us that we can indeed prevent cancer, as the majority of cancer cases are lifestyle and environmentally-related.

Modern science has found that a Mediterranean-style diet, combined with exercise and the non-use of tobacco, can prevent 70 percent of cancer. We know that lifestyle plays a major role in the prevention of cancer, which is why information like this is so important. We must begin to make healthy choices for ourselves and our children. In 2003, the American Cancer Society found that the heaviest people, in comparison to the leanest, had an increased death rate. Uterine cancer in women had a six-fold increase; liver cancer in men, a five-fold increase. Only about 10 percent of cancers are related to your genes.

This Biological Rejuvenation Program is about saving your life while, at the same time, giving you the highest genetic expression of health available to you right now. And just wait until you see the results you can achieve when you combine a Mediterranean diet, exercise and medical foods. You are going to love your body and your life!

Metabolic Syndrome Body Type

Earlier chapters of this book addressed insulin resistance, also known as metabolic syndrome. The devastation of this condition is so extensive that the body shape of someone with metabolic syndrome is going to be a combination of all the body types outlined above. This is because metabolic syndrome creates a loss of blood sugar regulation, which affects the entire endocrine system—including the thyroid gland, the adrenal gland and the reproductive hormones. The liver is vital to the stabilization of blood sugar and the conjugation of hormones. When the liver is stressed and inflammation occurs, this causes increased cholesterol and triglycerides, as well as the potential increase in C-reactive protein. If the liver continues to be increasingly stressed, it will become unable to handle its primary function of eliminating toxic metabolites in the body. This, in turn, creates an increase of metabolic toxins that circulate throughout the blood stream, causing joint aches and pains, swelling, water retention, lethargy and, truthfully, a foggy, half-lived life. Individuals with a *Metabolic Syndrome Body Type* have little to no internal spark.

It is my professional opinion (and has been scientifically proven), that insulin resistance is the underlying cause of many chronic health problems;

it creates the downward spiral of vitality that many people experience as they age. The problem is that many people have it, but few of them know it. As of January 2010 the US Department of Health and Human Services, National Institutes of Health stated that approximately 68 million or 25% of the US adult population has Metabolic Syndrome. Since Metabolic Syndrome is largely contributed to by high carbohydrate diets one can only imagine the number of children already suffering with this condition. Traditional medicine does not address it until it manifests as one of the multiple diseases it can create such as obesity, heart disease, diabetes, lifestyle related cancer and their multiple complications from these conditions such as renal failure, stroke, impotence etc. Remember, traditional medicine is the diagnosis and treatment of disease. For the medical community to become involved, you must have a disease that is diagnosable by their standards. Think about this: medical doctors believe that early detection is important, but early detection means you already have the disease! Integrative natural healthcare practitioners, by contrast, are committed to the prevention of disease. This does not make traditional medicine "wrong," only limited in its scope and ability to deliver truly effective healthcare, because its delivery system is only targeted toward disease care. Many of our most brilliant minds work in the field of traditional medicine (my husband included), and when you're sick, you may need them.

It is vitally important that we put forth an effort to prevent harmful lifestyle-related conditions, including metabolic syndrome. If we are successful in prevention, we may never need traditional medicine—except for emergency medicine (and this is where traditional medicine is really powerful). I just hope that none of us ever have to experience that power!

The really good news is that your lifestyle choices are entirely under your control. I created this *Fit, Fun and Fabulous* program so that you can better understand the importance of choosing wisely. As you begin to make different choices that detoxify the body, balance your hormones and get that insulin under control, you will notice an increase in vitality that will allow you to have the body you desire. You will feel truly alive, perhaps for the first time in a long time!

Chapter 10

TARGETED NUTRIENT SUPPORT

I often hear well-meaning, well-informed people say that they do not need to take vitamins and other supplements because they get all the nutrients they need in their food choices. I really wish this were the case, but it isn't. Allow me to explain why.

Since the 1930s, it has been proven that the soil in which our nation's food is grown is deficient in necessary nutrients. In 1936, the United States Senate was presented with the results of a scientific study that it had commissioned on the mineral content of our food. The study demonstrated that many of our diseases could be attributed to the fact that American soil no longer provided plants with the minerals that are so essential to human nourishment and nutritional health. This excerpt from Senate Document 264 of the 74th Congress was published in the March 1936 issue of *Cosmopolitan*: " ... 99 percent of the American people are deficient in ... minerals, and ... a marked deficiency in any one of the more important minerals actually results in disease."

If this were true in the 1930s, you can imagine what 80 additional years of industrial farming, herbicides and pesticides have done to our food sources. Even when we choose organic produce (and I hope you do), we still have to balance the deficit created from the depleted soil. Laboratory tests have proven that the fruits, vegetables, grains, eggs and meats of today are not what they were a few generations ago. The quality of milk that we consume today would not be adequate to sustain the life of a newborn calf, for example, and it is virtually impossible to eat enough fruits and vegetables to supply the body with the necessary mineral salts to achieve its optimal level of health. Vitamins are vital to our health, and each one of these complex biochemical substances is important for the normal functioning of our cells, tissue and bodily organs. When we are deficient in vitamins, disorders and diseases can occur. What you may not realize is that vitamins control the body's appropriation of minerals and, in the absence of minerals, vitamins have no function to perform. In other words, the body needs minerals in order for vitamins to be utilized.

In addition to poor soil quality, we also have excessive environmental and emotional stressors that our grandparents and great-grandparents didn't have to cope with. Of course, World Wars I and II and the Great Depression era were tremendously stressful. The truth is, every generation has had its share of stress to deal with, and our ability to survive as a human species is directly dependant upon our ability to adapt to our internal and external environments. Today's scientifically based nutrients help us with this adaptation process.

The Four Basic Nutrients

We don't live in a perfect world, because of our standard American dietary approaches, coupled with the depletion of nutrients in our soil, we are best served by first utilizing the 'basic four' nutritional protocols, which I will describe below:

1. A high-quality multivitamin, to fill in our nutritional gaps
2. High-quality antioxidants, to manage free radicals
3. Pure essential fatty acids (If you choose fish oils, make sure they are free of heavy metals and toxins.) To balance our omega 3's 6's and 9's
4a. For women, a whole bone supplement containing supportive nutrients such as calcium, magnesium, phosphorous, boron, vitamin K, vitamin D and other important minerals (Please note

that calcium taken without magnesium can create a magnesium deficiency which leads to constipation and depression; calcium carbonate is not an easily absorbed nutrient but is widely prescribed by unknowing medical physicians.) for skeletal strength.

4b. For men, prostate support to help offset the already outlined reproductive stressors from our environment

For the average person, it is nearly impossible to navigate the isles of nutritional supplements in health food stores and supermarkets in search of the best supplements, because the variety of choices can be overwhelming and many supplements are of inferior quality. Some stores and whole food markets have employees with a basic working knowledge of supplements, but I do not think it's wise to rely solely on their advice. The science of dietary supplementation has advanced so much during the past two decades, and my wish for you is to be able to take full advantage of these advancements while taking the least amount of supplements possible.

To understand how these nutrients can work together and which dietary supplements should be taken apart, on an empty stomach or with food, requires an enormous amount of education, monitoring and testing; this is best left to licensed natural healthcare providers and biochemists who dedicate their life to these studies.

What are Targeted Nutrients?

Sometimes we will have additional body stress due to illness, injury, overwork or difficult events in our lives. This is when target nutrients are helpful in addition to your basic four. Target nutrients are nutrients that have been clinically shown to be effective at addressing specific imbalances. For instance, resveratrol and vitamin E have been shown to support the cardiovascular system. Vitamins D, C and maitake mushrooms have been shown to support the immune system, especially when combined with probiotics. Hyaluronic acid, glucosamine and MSM are commonly known to support joint health. The B vitamins, when combined with dimethylglycine, can help with stress and can support learning. Turmeric and essential fatty acids can have a cooling effect on inflammation. In today's modern age, we are dealing with not only emotional and physical stressors, but also free-radical stress caused by environmental pollutants; these can be counterbalanced through high quality antioxidants, targeted liver support and targeted gut support. Our day-to-day emotional stress can be managed through "adaptogens," or herbs such a reishi mushroom, noni, ashwaganda, schisandra, gensing, holy basil, licorice and eleuthero, just to name a few, that clinically seem to have a normalizing effect on the body; they are capable of either toning down the activity of hyperfunctioning systems or strengthening the activity of hypofunctioning systems. These are excellent remedies to maintain balance. Immune weakness due to excess stress can be addressed through these adaptogens, as well as the probiotics and Vitamins D and C listed above.

Targeted nutrients are used to hone in on certain areas of the body that have been compromised for whatever reason—it could be environmental stressors that are affecting the thyroid gland, or leading a hectic lifestyle that ultimately affects the adrenal gland. It could be working in an industrial environment that taxes the liver, or the body's attempts to tolerate changes inherent in menopause that cause those uncomfortable hot flashes or seasonal changes that weaken many peoples immune system. This is why I have tried to create targeted nutrient groupings that incorporate the basic four while, at the same time, target specific challenges or meet specific needs, like supplements for vegetarians. These targeted nutrient groupings that I have created represent what I would call a general wellness outline. (Check them out in my online natural pharmacy at <drkathleenhartford.com>.)

* * *

There may be times when you want to complete a metabolic cleansing or detoxification protocol; this is something that I do twice a year. I also use a metabolic anti-inflammatory food every day that Dr Jeffery Bland PhD created called Inflammation 911 (available on my website). Osteoarthritis is very common in my family, and I do not want to leave myself open for any inflammatory processes. Inflammation 911 is a fully balanced meal replacement that I use as my breakfast. I also take menopausal support, because no level of discomfort is ok with me, and occasionally I take workout support for weightlifting. The best way to explore which targeted nutrients would be a right fit for you is to arrange for a nutritional coaching session with me or one of my coaches. Everybody is unique and that uniqueness will determine the most effective approach to targeted nutrients.

A "new you" is created every 11 months on the cellular level. The best way to guarantee that this renewed version of yourself is as healthy (or healthier) than the old you is to make sure your body has all of the nutrients it needs to generate healthy new cells, tissues and organs. Targeted supplementation will help ensure that these nutrients are available for a new, biologically younger, you!

WHERE TO BEGIN

Congratulations! You have just completed reading some of the most important information of your life, and for your life! Now comes the follow-through. Keep in mind that each topic covered in these chapters could be a book by itself (most already are!). My objective has been to distill the information into a workable explanation, so that you can understand the importance of each of these topics and apply them to your daily life.

One thing is certain: we are all going to age, at least chronologically. How we age is largely within our control. It is the result of the choices we make every day. Throughout this book, you have read snippets of results that our clients have gotten when utilizing the *Fit, Fun and Fabulous* program in their own lives. All of them have achieved these results in only 12 weeks. During those 12 weeks, these clients did several things by committing to this Biological Rejuvenation Program:

- they followed a Mediterranean-style diet that is naturally low in inflammatory food. (Visit www.fitfunandfabulous.com for a sample week of food ideas)
- they utilized the medical food called Inflammation 911 to further decrease systemic inflammation and improve their gut health (which directly affects immune health).
- they exercised three times a week using weight resistant exercise and other approaches that suited their lifestyle and

passions (visit <drkathleenhartford.com> for various exercise support).

- they maintained a journal that documented their daily activities, which helped them honor their agreement to themselves and define areas in which they may have been sabotaging their progress and utilized coaching from my staff to support their efforts.

Now that you have an awareness of the *Fit, Fun and Fabulous* program, you have power. Information is power—or should I say, information that is *applied* is powerful! I now invite you to be powerful in your life. Take control of your daily choices and allow yourself to achieve the highest level of health that is genetically available to you right here, right now. I promise you that the therapeutic effects of the program, when followed, will support you every day. Not only will you be *Fit and Fabulous*, you will have *Fun* while taking this journey toward reaching your fullest genetic potential for health and vitality. After all, what could be more enjoyable than watching you grow younger?

My hope is that you took advantage of the quick start guide at the beginning of this book and completed your biological age assessment. Every 12 weeks, I'd like you to do another assessment to make certain that you stay on track. If you follow the program, you will indeed become biologically younger and should experience that change in all areas of your life—inside, as well as your outward appearance. My hope is that once you experience the benefits of the *Fit Fun & Fabulous Life* you will incorporate this 12-week program as a way of life.

Here's the deal: no matter what you take on in life, you will have good days and bad days. At times you will follow the program beautifully, but at other times you will ask, What program? This is why we are available to you as coaches. The program itself is simple, but it's not always easy to change ingrained lifestyle behaviors. If it were as effortless as providing a lifestyle change program with no ongoing support, there would not be thousands of weight-loss programs out there and hundreds of thousand of people that have lost weight through them only to gain the weight back again. This is why we offer personal coaching sessions, online resources and multiple teleseminars—to be your support and to help you stay on track.

Consider Personal Coaching for Ongoing Support

The concept of coaching has been around since the human race began. Elders have always counseled the young. Masters in all art forms have taken on promising apprentices, and there isn't a world-class athlete who does not rely on the expertise of a coach. In short, a coach is someone who:

- Supports you where you are.
- Listens to where you would like to be.
- Helps sharpen your focus.
- Gives advice, counsel and support based on their experience and knowledge of who you are.

A coach's job is to chunk your challenges down and bring important areas of potential breakthroughs to your awareness. Awareness is the beginning of all conscious living. Awareness of these areas gives you the chance to explore where you are, who you are and how you want to BE in the world. It's exciting, it's juicy and it would be an honor for our coaching team to support you through your physical, spiritual and emotional journey called life.

Your Most Noble Purpose

Now, I want to be very real and one-on-one with you. I love teaching people not only about the importance of health, but also how they can maintain their health and vitality for a lifetime. I enjoy this process because I understand that we must first have a healthy foundation, a body that feels good and a body that frees us from health worries so that we can get on with, what I believe is, our true purpose in life.

Our most noble purpose is to achieve self-realization, to truly, deeply and passionately know ourselves. We cannot do this in a half-dead body. We cannot do this worrying from one doctor visit to the next. We can only do this when our energy is high, our bodies are running like well-tuned sports cars, and our minds are clear of fog and free of the worries that come from the lack of ease (dis-ease) and function of our bodies.

When we integrate our wellness approaches through supporting the mind, body and spirit, the body has to come first. The next step, the mind, will by far be our greatest lifetime challenge. Once we master the mind—including our thought processes and our limited thinking—we can then create a spiritual life, one in which we are in service to the world. (Your world may be your family, your customers or the entire planet.) In my world, I find that it is important to know yourself, your values, your true heart's desires and your passions—or, you will continue to mis-create your life, leaving yourself empty, hopeless and feeling like a failure.

I extend to you an invitation to truly explore your passions and create a life based on your values and heart's desires. We host retreats that will help you to do just that. Whether you have 30 minutes for a telephone coaching session, five hours for a half-day rejuvenation retreat, or four days and a big heart for an intensive retreat, we are here for you. We even run free teleseminars to help keep you engaged and focused. For more information on all of these offerings, visit <drkathleenhartford.com>.

Ideally, I would love to meet you in person and work with you one-on-one. If you are in the Pittsburgh area or would like to travel to our office for a visit, simply call 1 (800) 893-5000. Our office is called the Health Pyramid Longevity and Vitality Center and is located about 25 miles northeast of Pittsburgh. We would be honored to help balance your physical body with structural, biochemical, bio-energetic and emotional support. To learn more about our bodywork offerings, visit <healthpyramid.com>.

Whatever your next step is, we are committed to supporting you through your process. Thank you so much for "investing in your life" with me!

APPENDIX

THE 12 BIOMARKERS OF AGING

- **BIOMARKER 1:** *Muscle Age Based on Body Cell Mass and Muscle Mass*

Your muscle age is based on the percentage of lean muscle in your body composition. We lose an average of 6.2 pounds of muscle each decade over the age of 18. Once we reach age 45, this rate accelerates. I don't know about you, but I can't think of many people who have lost weight since high school. Unless you have been actively participating in some form of weight-resistant or muscle-building exercise, you have lost lean muscle every decade since then. So let's say you've gained 15 pounds since high school and lost 6.2 pounds of muscle in each of the two decades since graduating: you now have accumulated 12.4 (6.2 x 2 decades) plus 15 pounds, a total of 27.4 pounds of fat tissue. If you didn't gain a pound yet have not maintained your lean muscle mass through weight-resistant exercise, you would still have lost 6.2 pounds of lean muscle mass per decade. This means that you have 12.4 more fat pounds making up your body composition than you did in high school.

Fat is not inert tissue simply sitting there as stored energy; it is highly inflammatory in nature and complications from its inflammatory nature emerge due to the immune/metabolic relationship. This immune/metabolic component is vital when understanding the devastating health effects of excessive fat tissue, and speaks to many of the new auto-immune diseases we see today.

Fat tissue is made up of adipose cells, which increase in size but not number. As we deposit more fat tissue into the adipose cells, these cells produce something called cytokines—small, secreted proteins that, among other things, produce and regulate immunities and inflammation. When adipose cells grow larger, they produce more cytokines, leading to more inflammation and a greater challenge for your immune system.

Weight loss through a low-inflammatory diet and exercise will improve the situation. Several studies have confirmed that as overweight people lose weight through the simple (though not necessarily easy) lifestyle changes outlined in this Biological Rejuvenation Program, those inflammation-producing cytokines are reduced and numerous health measures improve. These improvements are clinically proven through, not just weight loss, but changes in blood pressure, blood fats, blood sugar and other parameters. In fact, this Biological Rejuvenation Program will help you achieve the results in 12 weeks, that normally take two years, through diet alone.

Allow me to take a minute to address weight loss programs that do not monitor body composition—that is, the tissue that composes your body, focusing on fat, water and muscle. In my opinion, such programs are misleading. Unless you are monitoring the type of tissue that you're losing in your weight loss endeavors, how do you know if you are experiencing healthy weight loss, which is actually *fat* loss? Anybody can lose pounds. But if the diet you are on is causing a breakdown of muscle in order to stabilize your plummeting blood sugar, thereby creating gluconeogenesis (meaning, you are making new glucose from your muscle tissue), then your weight loss is from muscle loss. This is very unhealthy, it will also decrease your basal metabolic rate (see Biomarker 3), thereby making it harder for you to lose any body fat at all.

As another example, if you lose water weight (yes, you have lost pounds), the weight will return once you rehydrate or resume unhealthy lifestyle habits. Some weight loss plans are based on calculating your body mass index (BMI), but this alone will not provide you with adequate body composition information. It is simply a height-and-weight calculation. So if you are experiencing sarcopenia or are a skinny fat person (thin body with a high percentage of fat tissue, very common in our elderly population), you will be misled into thinking that you are healthy.

So as you can see, healthy weight loss is fat loss, and fat loss is easily influenced by two factors:

- Level of purposeful physical activity
- Biochemical balance through nutrition

To maintain and maximize fat burning, muscle function and overall health, we must have a supportive nutritional plan, one that favors healthy hormone balance, especially in relation to balancing blood sugar. The good news is that studies show that with the right type and amount of exercise, individuals in their 60s, 70s, 80s, and even 90s can improve their muscle strength and size the same as younger adults. Speaking of muscle mass, this directly correlates to the second biomarker of aging.

- **BIOMARKER 2:** *Strength and Musculoskeletal Fitness*

Building muscle tissue and regaining or maintaining strength obviously go hand in hand. The muscles that attach to and move the skeleton are referred to as "skeletal muscles." These muscles receive direction from the motor nerves that run from your central nervous system via the spinal cord and its branches, which exit from the spinal column (one of the most important reasons to participate in chiropractic care). These sets of motor nerves and the muscle fibers that they supply are known as "motor units."

The body has two types of muscle fibers: red and white. Red muscle fibers are called "slow twitch" or "low force" fibers, and they are activated during activities that occur over time. They are most active during endurance activities such as swimming and long-distance running. White muscle fibers are "fast twitch," high intensity fibers. They are used during activities like lifting and sprinting. Any activity that occurs with bursts of energy would fall into this group; the muscle creates a quick contraction but also fatigues quickly.

Typically, we lose 20 percent of our motor units between the ages of 30 and 70. Motor units are a single-motor neuron and all of the muscle fibers it innervates. This is how the nervous system controls and coordinates your movements. How does this 20 percent loss occur? The same way that we lose muscle mass: what you don't use, you lose. We typically stop challenging not just our muscles but also our balance/proprioception (our ability to sense the position, location, orientation and movement of the body and its parts). This contributes to the loss of coordinated movement. At first it's subtle. We are not able to do things we used to do, or do them as well. We notice a loss of "muscle memory." As time goes on, our gait begins to change as we widen our stance to maintain our balance. Over time, we become vulnerable to falls and fractures as our 10th biomarker, bone mineral density, diminishes, as well.

We also lose about 30 percent of our muscle cells between the ages of 20 and 70. The loss of both muscle cells and muscle mass adversely affects so many areas of our health, including:

- Decreased blood sugar tolerance
- Declining metabolism
- Increased body fat
- Reduced aerobic capacity
- Loss of bone mineral density

Sounds like a bit of a bummer, right? Well only if you are a committed couch potato. Remember, studies prove that with the right exercise, individuals in their sixth, seventh, eighth and even ninth decade of life can expect improvements in strength and muscle cell size comparable to younger people doing the same amount of exercise. For women, this is especially good news in the area of osteoporosis (which we will address in Biomarker 10). This is why so much emphasis is given to physical activity and strength training in this Biological Rejuvenation Program!

Look at it this way: Yes, your skeletal muscles are like your body's engine and your skeleton is the chassis. The more efficient your engine, the farther your chassis will take you. The higher the octane—that is, the "cleaner" your food—the more efficiently you will burn this fuel. Your body can be a sleek, turbo-charged Corvette or a dinky, rusted out pick-up truck ... it's your choice.

This loss of muscle mass also translates into a decline in our third biomarker.

- **BIOMARKER 3:** *Basal Metabolic Rate*

Your basal metabolic rate, or BMR, is the rate at which your body burns calories while at rest. Your body expends energy 24/7. It takes energy to breathe and talk, for your heart to beat, even to sleep. Your BMR is like your body's engine while idling at a red light. Exercise is analogous to stepping on the gas once the light turns green. Your muscles require fuel to move. The more muscle mass you have, the more fuel (calories) is required to feed them. So I ask the question again: Is your body a sporty "muscle" car or a dilapidated pick-up truck?

If you have not been maintaining your lean muscles mass, you've probably noticed that every year it becomes harder to eat whatever you want and stay slim. In fact, you are probably eating the same way you always have, but suddenly you are putting on weight. Unfortunately, our BMR decreases as we age. If we are losing 6.2 pounds of muscle every decade, then it's understandable why we can no longer eat what we used to eat. We don't have the same muscle mass to demand the food and burn the calories, and all those unused calories are neatly stored as body fat.

Depriving yourself of food with the hope of losing weight decreases your BMR. The body, in its infinite survival wisdom, adapts to a decrease in calories and lowers its BMR to conserve fuel. When the body begins to conserve its fuel, it also begins to deposit fat for the long haul; this is what it's programmed to do in case of starvation. When we do not eat regularly or when we diminish our caloric intake to the point of destabilizing our delicate levels of glucose (blood sugar), the body will conserve that fat and efficiently digest your muscles for blood sugar stabilization. Yes, it becomes catabolic. It breaks down tissue in order to support survival.

Right about now, you're probably ready for some positive news, so here it is: you can increase your BMR through proper exercise and nutrition. A regular routine of cardiovascular exercise or consistent weight training to increase muscle mass can increase your BMR, thereby improving your fitness and lowering your biological age.

If the muscle in your body is your body's "engine" and muscle requires calories, then the more muscle your have, the more calories that will be required to fuel that muscle. This means that you can enjoy more calories and not gain weight! As we age and lose muscle mass, however, our engine slows down and we require fewer calories. Unfortunately, few of us tend to eat less as we age, so weight gain is an inevitable consequence. All the more reason to improve your BMR with muscle building activities, exercise and a healthy diet consisting of:

- Lean proteins
- Organic vegetables
- Whole grains (provided you are not wheat intolerant)
- Fruits

- **BIOMARKER 4:** *Body Fat Percentage*

Body fat is pretty much the inversion of Biomarker 1, body cell mass. In Biomarker 1, we are most interested in determining your lean muscle mass, or the percentage of your body that is muscle tissue. As Biomarker 1 goes down, Biomarker 4 typically goes up. Your body fat percentage typically increases as you age. A sedentary person will have about twice the body fat as they had in their late teens and twenties.

Unless we are actively maintaining our lean muscle mass and following a healthy dietary lifestyle, we cannot avoid this downward spiral. Two-thirds of Americans are overweight and one-third of them are obese. This has created an epidemic of high blood pressure, atherosclerosis (hardening of the arteries), heart disease, heart-related deaths, strokes and diabetes. Many types of cancer have also been linked to obesity.

This may surprise you: thin people can also have excessive fat. Body fat cannot always be "seen" and, for this reason, it can be deceiving. To the eye, you may appear to be thin, but a bioimpedence analysis or body composition scan of your body mass may reveal that you have a high percentage of fat tissue. This is why it is important to use a fat measuring device instead of the typical Body Mass Index based simply on your height and weight. Unless you get a proper reading on your percentage of body fat, you will not be able to monitor and ensure that you are losing "fat" pounds.

As previously mentioned, almost all weight loss programs can demonstrate weight loss, but those that do not monitor fat loss are dangerous and misleading; you may think you're getting healthier, but a skinny "high body fat percentage" person who is experiencing sarcopenia—age-related muscle loss and strength—is still at risk for disease and accelerated aging. In the past, it was believed that fat tissue was largely inert and was simply an energy storage facility to be called upon during times of caloric shortage or when extra energy was being expended. I'm certain that this is how God intended for it to work during times of starvation or food shortages. It is now known, however, that numerous biochemical reactions occur within fat tissue that cause systemic inflammation. In other words, the body very wisely utilizes fat as a storage area for environmental toxins, excess hormones and a host of other nasty substances that are best kept away from sensitive tissue and organs. Most of these things (especially those from our environment) have changed dramatically since the dawn of time. The amount of toxins that your body is now asked to process—many of which end up deposited in your fat tissues—is killing us through inflammation.

It is vital to verify that your weight loss is coming from fat loss. If not, you run the risk of creating the disease of aging mentioned above called sarcopenia. The first characteristic of this is a decrease in muscle size; the cause is often unknown or accepted as normal aging, weakness and frailty. With sarcopenia, muscle fibers are replaced with fat tissue (inflammatory tissue) and an increase in fibrosis. Fibrotic tissue is "akinetic," meaning that it lacks motion. This contributes greatly to a loss of flexibility and an increase of tissue pain as we age and continue to lose muscle mass.

As explained with Biomarker 3, your BMR also decreases as your muscle mass decreases and your fat increases. This begins a rapid acceleration in the aging process for multiple reasons—the most important of which is the inflammatory nature of fat tissue.

Fat is more than an aesthetic concern. Fat is very active and destructive tissue, filled with those pesky cytokines that contribute greatly to inflammation and many of the disease processes we find today. In the body this translates to an accelerated aging process found even in our children, making us biologically years older than our chronological ages.

Fat, particularly around your waist, raises your risk of serious health issues such as:

- Diabetes
- Heart disease
- Many forms of cancer
- Insomnia
- Musculoskeletal and joint stress
- Osteoporosis and osteopenia, even in children
- The emotional toll of obesity and the inability to actively participate in life with peers and family

Overweight? You're Not Alone

Obesity has created an epidemic of health issues that can do more than just shorten your life. Obesity-related poor health forces you to deal with the emotional and physical stress caused by disease and suffering. It can create misery in your life, instead of allowing you to live with joy and purpose.

Medical science acknowledges that inflammation is the root cause of many serious diseases—including diabetes, heart disease and chronic immune system dysfunction. Whether that immune dysfunction creates a recurrent condition such as seasonal bronchitis or a diagnosis of any of our newly discovered disease states such as fibromyalgia or chronic fatigue. It is important to look at the broad picture to determine what causes and contributes to inflammatory conditions. It's not just the food you eat but also the water you drink, the air your breathe, the type of exercise you do and even your thoughts. The mind and the body are very integrated and, for this reason, we must maintain a daily awareness of the physical and emotional patterns that ultimately influence and direct our lives.

- **BIOMARKER 5:** *Body Fat Distribution*

The distribution of body fat (where your fat is held) is especially important to your health. People who hold weight around their waist— what is typically referred to as the "apple" shape—are at much greater risk of developing heart disease, stroke and diabetes. In order to monitor the risk factors in relation to one's biological age, a waist-to-hip ratio is taken. This ratio is an important health assessment indicator.

Carrying body fat around the midsection indicates the serious condition we discussed in Chapter 4 called metabolic syndrome. This is a pre-diabetic condition that consists of a cluster of symptoms that occur together: elevated blood pressure and insulin levels, excess body fat around the waist and abnormal cholesterol levels. Any of these symptoms can occur independently and create a serious disease risk; when they appear in combination, however, your risk of heart disease, stroke or diabetes is even greater.

According to a national health survey, more than one in five Americans have metabolic syndrome. The number of people who have it increases with age; so while the accelerated aging process can begin in our youth, it affects more than 40 percent of people in their 60s and 70s in the form of metabolic syndrome. The most effective way to address, and even reverse, metabolic syndrome or any of its components is ... you guessed it! ... through the simple lifestyle changes outlined in this Biological Rejuvenation Program. I can't stress enough that this program is truly the healthiest and best way to delay and even prevent the development of serious health problems.

Could You Have Metabolic Syndrome?

If you have three or more of the following indicators, you may be dealing with metabolic syndrome.

- Waistline of 40 inches or more for men, and 35 inches or more for women (measured across the belly)
- Blood pressure of 130/85 mm Hg or higher, or taking blood pressure medication
- Triglyceride level above 150 mg/dl
- Fasting blood glucose (sugar) level greater than 100 mg/dl, or taking glucose lowering medication
- High density lipoprotein level (HDL) less than 40 mg/dl for men, or under 50 mg/dl for women

Who is Most at Risk for Metabolic Syndrome?

- People with central obesity (increased fat in the abdomen and waist)
- People with diabetes mellitus or a strong family history of it
- People with other clinical features of "insulin resistance" such as skin changes like acanthosis nigricans (or, "dirty skin" on the back of the neck or underarms) or skin tags (usually on the neck)
- People with a triglyceride to HDL cholesterol ratio of > 3

What are the Symptoms of Metabolic Syndrome?

Usually, there are no immediate physical symptoms. Medical problems associated with metabolic syndrome develop over time and most people are not aware that they have it. Medical doctors don't readily diagnose it until diseases created from prolonged metabolic syndrome are expressed. Our goal with this program is to reverse the condition of metabolic syndrome *before* diseases begin to appear. You can be assured that, even if you are already suffering with diseases associated with metabolic syndrome, this program can improve those conditions and even, in many cases, reverse them.

What is the Cause and How Can Metabolic Syndrome be Prevented or Reversed?

While the exact cause of metabolic syndrome is not known, it seems to have several causes that work together over time to create the syndrome, and many of its features are associated with "insulin resistance." This means that the body is not able to use insulin efficiently to lower glucose and triglyceride levels. Insulin resistance is a combination of genetic and lifestyle factors such as diet, physical fitness, chronic stress and even interrupted sleep patterns, like sleep apnea and menopausal insomnia.

Since a high-insulin lifestyle is the main underlying factor for metabolic syndrome, it's important to create a lifestyle that balances your blood sugar and maintains a healthy cell wall for nutrients to travel through. How is this achieved? Here are some really good guidelines, all of which we've already covered in the chapters of this book.

- Eat a Mediterranean-style diet of whole, plant-based food
- Engage in physical activity that creates lean muscle mass
- Eat frequent, balanced meals to avoid hunger and low blood sugar
- Reduce the use of stimulants and other serotonin-releasing simple carbohydrates, such as white bread, bagels, etc.
- Incorporate effective stress management skills into your life to control cortisol levels
- Use high-quality target nutrients to offset the micro-nutrient deficiencies in food due to depleted soil content and lack of sun exposure
- Balance hormones and eliminate environmental stressors that create hormonal stress (for more on this, read Chapter 7)

As you incorporate these health-enhancing changes into your life, you will lose weight. Healthy weight loss comes from having a healthy lifestyle!

- **BIOMARKER 6:** *Aerobic Capacity*

Aerobic capacity refers to your body's ability to take in and properly utilize oxygen. For your aerobic capacity to be high, you must have healthy lungs, a strong heart and an efficient circulatory system. Efficiency in any activity comes from repetitive use so, yes, to increase your aerobic capacity, you must exercise the heart and create efficiency within your circulatory system.

The term "VO2 max" refers to the maximum amount of oxygen (in milliliters) that one can use in one minute per kilogram of body weight. Those who are fit have higher VO2 max values and can exercise more intensely than those who are not as well conditioned. Numerous studies show that you can increase your VO2 max by working out at an intensity that raises your heart rate to between 65 and 85 percent of its maximum capacity for at least 20 minutes three to five times a week.

Factors That Affect VO2 Max

Typically, aerobic capacity declines with age. Men peak at about 20 years of age while woman typically peak at about age 30. I say "typically" because, as with the other biomarkers, aerobic capacity can be improved with regular exercise and nutrition. Returning to the VO2 max of our youth takes longer as we get older, but is well worth the effort. It not only improves our biological age but also our ability to participate in the world with our friends and family doing the things that we love.

I personally enjoy interval training, which involves a variety of exercises that can be performed right at home at any age. Many excellent books have been written about interval training, and specific exercises may be recommended based on your age and purpose. My nephews' interval training for college football, for example, is different from the interval training routine that I follow to maintain my health. I try to keep pace with them, but I usually end up on the floor begging for mercy. Interesting though … they are still afraid of me when I box!

- **BIOMARKER 7:** *Blood Sugar Tolerance*
Blood sugar (glucose) tolerance is your body's ability to withstand blood sugar in the blood stream. For most people, aging is synonymous with an increase in blood sugar levels because of our high insulin lifestyles. This compromised ability to regulate and utilize glucose is quite common. The first sign of trouble is often weight gain around the midsection, fatigue and ultimately, if left unchecked, diabetes. Unfortunately, blood tests can detect this problem only after it has become pathological. By that time, damage has already occurred and it's more difficult to regain your health; so it's important to maintain balanced blood sugar levels and avoid the downward spiral of premature aging.

Remember how we said that your body is continually adapting to your choices and your environment? Well, insulin is a hormone that responds to the type of food you ingest. It regulates fat metabolism and controls blood sugar. Blood sugar has a very narrow range through which it can fluctuate and be healthy. If it goes too low, it creates a condition known as hypoglycemia, or low blood sugar; if it goes too high, it creates a condition called hyperglycemia. Initially most people fluctuate between these two. It is what Dr. Victor Frank, the creator of the Total Body Modification Technique, called "oppositic." Think of the children who enter school bouncing off the walls from their sugary breakfast cereals, then can't keep their eyes open to focus on their studies by 10 o'clock. (This is why the 10 a.m. coffee break became popular.) Proper exercise, improved nutrition and the right nutritional supplement program can result in marked improvement in blood sugar tolerance and balance.

Proper dietary changes (see the list of *Glycemic Foods* in the Appendix) begin to balance the crucial glucose-regulating hormones, while increased exercise lowers insulin resistance and improves the cells' ability to utilize the sugars that are present—thus avoiding metabolic syndrome, or insulin resistance.

I rarely pass up a piece of Hartford birthday cake when celebrating with my family. (Okay, the recipe comes out of a box, but it is so good!) The key is to not overindulge. I believe it was Dr. Deepak Chopra whom I first heard say, "Everything in moderation, including moderation." As you create a sense of awareness about your body, you will no longer enjoy the way you feel after excessive indulgence in high-calorie food or alcohol. Chances are you will probably feel a bit bloated and "yucky" after eating a piece of cake or indulging in too much of anything. Your increased awareness will support you toward making better choices again and again. On the other hand, if you participate in a "high insulin lifestyle" (as many Americans do), that is a different story. Science has proven that these habits will harm you over the long haul:

- Poorly balanced, high carbohydrate meals
- Skipping meals, especially breakfast
- Lack of proper exercise
- Repetitive use of stimulants, soda, sugar, caffeine and energy drinks
- Lack of quality sleep
- Lack of stress management
- Micronutrient imbalance (refer to Chapter 10 for more on this)
- Hormonal imbalance (Remember, insulin is a hormone.)

When we participate in these health-diminishing habits we create hyperinsulinemia—an excess circulation of insulin through the body due to an overload of sugar in the diet or a lifestyle that increases cellular resistance to the insulin receptors on the cell wall. Excess insulin creates increased fat deposits, which in turn create increased inflammation. Prolonged inflammation contributes to the creation of pain and disease processes in the body. If we continue with these health-diminishing activities, we will become insulin resistant on the cellular level. This means that the body will begin to shut down insulin receptor sites on the cell membranes to protect the body from sugar overload. Insulin resistance leads to the release of more insulin as the body attempts to lower blood sugar levels in the blood stream. When this is left unchecked, the pancreas eventually burns out and can no longer respond to the body's need for insulin. The result? The onset of Type 2 diabetes and a continued increase in fat deposits throughout the body, especially around the mid-section. There is another connection with diabetes relationship to Alzheimer's disease, which science is just now discovering. It is known that diabetics have a 65 percent increased risk of being diagnosed with Alzheimer's disease, which was not really understood until now. Scientists are now discovering that your brain makes it's own insulin to convert the glucose in your blood stream into the food it needs to survive. When your brain cells become insulin resistant and the production of insulin begins to diminish, parts of your brain virtually starve as it is deprived of the glucose converted energy it needs especially for memory. Increased insulin concentrations (due to cell wall resistance) also appear to boost levels of beta-amyloid, a protein involved in the formation of senile plaques that can lead to Alzheimer's.

Fat—which, as we've said, is a major source of silent inflammation—is filled with cytokinese and arachodonic acid, which is a precursor to pain and inflammation. The higher your insulin levels, the more your body is stimulated to increase levels of arachodonic acid. The more pain and inflammation we have, the harder it is to exercise; the harder it is to exercise, the more weight we put on. So many Americans find themselves caught in this vicious cycle day after day. What is truly frightening is that, as adults and parents, we are allowing this to also become prevalent in our children.

It is predicted that one-third of children born in the year 2000 will become diabetic—not *might* or *could*, but *will*. Given the current state of our healthcare economy, how will these children be cared for as they enter early adulthood already racked with pain, heart disease, loss of limbs and all of the other diseases that obesity and diabetes influence? It is our duty to care for our children and the younger generations in a responsible way by modeling good health ourselves and providing healthy foods and environments for those we love.

- **BIOMARKER 8:** *Cholesterol / HDL Ratio*

We've been hearing a lot about cholesterol, but what exactly is it? Cholesterol is a fatty substance created by your liver. Your body needs it for hormone balancing, eyesight and … yes, to fight inflammation, if needed. It also plays an essential role in the health of your cell membranes and sex hormone metabolism.

There is some confusion about cholesterol, so let's set the record straight. First of all, it is not an "essential nutrient," because your body manufactures it whenever necessary. Cholesterol circulates in the bloodstream as "lipoproteins," or combinations of fats bound to proteins. Some cholesterol-containing lipoproteins have been found to actually protect us from heart disease; these are called high-density lipoproteins, or HDLs. The other type of lipoproteins—called low density (LDL) and very low density (VLDL) are the ones associated with arteriosclerosis, or hardening of the arteries. Studies indicate that when the ratio of total cholesterol over HDL cholesterol is 4.5 or lower, there is a reduced risk of heart and circulatory disease. Unfortunately, cholesterol/HDL ratios typically elevate with age, thereby increasing your risk of disability, premature aging and death.

It is believed that this elevation in cholesterol is due to a corresponding increase in acidity and—once again—that ever pesky inflammation in the body. As inflammation increases, the risk of this inflammation "pitting" the arteriole wall is heightened. To protect the arteriole wall from this destructive pitting, your body releases cholesterol, which acts as a sticky adhesive "band aid" type substance. The cholesterol adheres to the artery wall to strengthen the pitted areas caused by inflammation.

As you can see, the body is creating a perfect response to a potentially damaging condition. That's a good thing but, as with most things, too much of it can turn bad. Saying that cholesterol causes heart disease is like saying grey hair makes you old. Cholesterol itself is not the culprit—inflammation is. If you want to lower your cholesterol levels, you must address the inflammatory process in the body so the liver can chill and stop producing high levels of cholesterol. This is why the Biological Rejuvenation Program includes anti-inflammatory food that, along with stress management approaches, will directly affect your cholesterol HDL ratio—read this carefully—with *no adverse side effects*. One very important *positive* side effect, of course, is a dramatically healthier cardiovascular system.

Clearly, the key to reducing LDLs (the most harmful form of cholesterol) and raising HDLs (the beneficial form) is a combination of better dietary management, proper supplementation and a consistent exercise program. Dietary changes alone can lower LDLs, but it takes both exercise and a reduction in body fat to raise HDLs.

What is both interesting and paradoxical here is that for some people to reduce body fat, they must actually increase their intake of "healthy" fats and oils. One of the greatest dietary lies sold to the American public is the concept of the "low-fat carbohydrate," which is really slow death in the guise of a healthy food. Twenty years ago I stated that triglycerides would soon become as big a health concern as cholesterol. If you want your triglycerides to go through the roof, eat low-fat carbohydrates; if you want your body fat to increase, eat low-fat carbohydrates. This can be confusing because you may think "low fat" is good but, in the form of *processed* carbohydrates, it is not good. Again, I can't stress enough how important it is to eat food, as much as possible, in its natural form, the way God made it.

- **BIOMARKER 9:** *Blood Pressure*

Hypertension, often referred to as "the silent killer," affects 65 million Americans by increasing their risk of heart attacks, stroke and other serious diseases. What is hypertension? Basically, your blood pressure has two components:

- Systolic pressure (read first) reflects the pressure on your arteries when your heart contracts.

- Diastolic pressure (read second) represents the pressure in your arteries between heartbeats when your heart is at rest.

Normal blood pressure is less than 140 systolic (with 120 considered ideal) and less than 85 diastolic. Even though some people are genetically predisposed to hypertension, a proper nutrition and exercise program will restore normal healthy pressures in nearly everyone. Various medical studies indicate that a major culprit of high blood pressure may be inflammation. (I hope you are now beginning to see the connection between inflammation and just about every biomarker being discussed here!) As previously mentioned, I believe that over the next decade we will find that most diseases—from cancer to heart disease—are related to the body's inflammatory response to an unhealthy environment and lifestyle choices related to food, stress, drugs and excessive alcohol.

Inflammation worsens with age because, if we don't address it and make the appropriate lifestyle changes, its effect is cumulative. In fact, our lifestyle usually becomes more inflammatory with age as we become more sedentary, eat richer food and take on increased stress. None of our disease processes occur overnight, but rather over time as we continue to participate in health-destroying habits.

We can also have blood pressure that is too low, the symptoms of which are very similar to those of low blood sugar levels: episodes of weakness and light-headedness, especially with sudden changes of posture called postural hypotension. In more chronic cases, this hypotension—particularly if it is posture-related—can be a sign of adrenal insufficiency and the result of prolonged distress. If this is suspected, further tests on adrenal function should be done. Conducting blood pressure tests in several different postures can be a valuable screening tool here. Most often, once you stand for a second, postural hypotension will normalize and you will feel fine, but it is not normal; your body is telling you that it needs support. Simple supplements that bolster your adrenal glad function can address this condition quite easily and safely.

Hypotension can also be related to dehydration and electrolyte imbalances following heavy exercise in very warm weather or after protracted vomiting or diarrhea. If you have been ill and vomiting for prolonged periods of time, you could be at great risk of severe dehydration. Please be certain to get plenty of fluids or consult a physician if you have been too sick to do so.

Sub-clinical dehydration is a very common state that I find in many patients. This alone can cause headaches, pain, constipation and sluggishness. I ask my patients to drink two-thirds of an ounce of water for each pound of body weight. The calculation is:

.66 x your weight = optimum purified water intake in ounces

- **BIOMARKER 10:** *Bone Mineral Density*

There is typically an age-related decline in bone mineral density that leaves older adults with weakened bones and at risk of disability and life-threatening complications. I say "typically" because it seems to be related to a sedentary lifestyle that no longer includes weight-loading the spine during purposeful exercise. The latter stages of bone mineral loss are called "osteoporosis." Yes, osteoporosis is accelerated in menopausal women but, contrary to popular belief, it affects men, too. Peak bone density is reached between the ages of 28 and 35 in men and women; studies show that, thereafter, bone mineral density typically declines by one percent each year.

This condition is beginning at an earlier age in current generations of children, due to lifestyle habits that create acidity and inflammation in the body. The acid/alkaline balance in your bloodstream is critical in maintaining healthy bones. What makes this a challenging area for teens and young adults is their excessive consumption of carbonated soft drinks and sugary so-called energy drinks.

If you are eating mostly an inflammatory "acid ash" diet, your body will leach calcium from your bones to neutralize the acidity. "Acidic" in this context doesn't refer to the pH of the food (such as oranges), but rather the pH of the "ash," which is the substance left when food is metabolized by the body. "Acid ash" foods are meats, processed carbohydrates, soft drinks and sweets. By contrast, fruits and vegetables are alkaline foods (refer to the *Acid and Alkaline Food Indexes* in the Appendix). When you start to push the level toward an acidic pH, the body will respond by releasing a very effective buffer; unfortunately, that buffer is calcium from your bones. When this buffering process goes on for years, it diminishes the density of the bone, leaving you osteopenic or osteoporotic.

Something called Wolff's Law is also at play here. It states: "If the loading on a bone decreases, the bone will become weaker due to turnover. [*Remember, you create a new skeleton every 11 months.*] It is less metabolically costly to maintain and there is no stimulus for continued remodeling that is required to maintain bone mass." In other words, what you don't use, you lose. So, to maintain healthy bone density, eat an alkaline plant-based diet and do weight resistance exercise.

Osteoporosis is not determined by age or menopause but rather is preventable through diet and exercise. Without weight resistance exercise and an alkaline plant-based diet, however, postmenopausal women are more at risk. After menopause, typical bone loss increases two to three percent per year; for some, it can be as high as 15 percent. The worst thing that women can do is to follow a doctor's advice to take calcium supplements alone. Calcium alone does not enhance bone growth; in fact, when taken on its own, it will create a magnesium deficiency, leaving a woman constipated, depressed and with deeply sore muscles. This targeted nutrient component must include adequate levels of associated bone building nutrients, not just calcium. (Refer to Chapter 10 for more on targeted nutrients.)

It may shock you to learn that your rate of bone loss increases 50-fold during prolonged bed rest. Research shows that two weeks of bed rest can cause as much bone loss as one full year of aging! Once again, as with the previous biomarkers, the very best prescription for the prevention and treatment of bone loss is supportive nutrition and proper exercise, particularly in the form of weight-resistant exercise. Wolff's Law states that bone matrix (new bone) is deposited in the bone in direct proportion to the amount of stress placed on the bone. If we are not stressing the bone with purposeful movement and weight resistance, the body no longer sees a need to strengthen its skeletal structure. It is important to monitor this before you become osteoporitic.

As with most biomarkers, there is a simple test, which many alternative health care practitioners utilize, to assess whether you are losing significant bone density. It involves an analysis of your urine to determine the levels of byproducts of bone breakdown; when elevated, these byproducts can signal an accelerated loss of bone. Corrective measures can then be initiated and a re-test done several weeks later to ensure resolution of the condition.

- **Biomarker 11:**   *Internal Temperature Regulation*

The human body is able to actively regulate its internal temperature somewhere between 98°F (36.6°C) and 100°F (37.7°C), in spite of various forces that act to cool off the body. This "temperature control" operates through a region of the brain called the hypothalamus, which contains the mechanisms to sense and monitor the body's internal temperature. As we age, our body's ability to regulate our internal temperature declines. Our thermoregulatory systems begin to struggle with changes in our external environment. Both cold and hot weather become more of a problem and can actually pose a danger to the elderly.

A complex set of factors is responsible for these difficulties; it is a delicate dance, beginning with skin sensors that communicate with the hypothalamus and the glands of the endocrine system. Two very important factors in this communication process are proper hydration and electrolyte balance, especially with respect to adapting to hot weather. This can be helped dramatically with proper nutrition and coaching on the quality and quantity of beverages consumed. (Remember to drink .66 times your body weight in ounces of water each day.) Another factor that directly affects thermoregulation is the status of the body's essential micronutrients; this is particularly important in helping the body adapt to colder environments. Insufficiency of iodine or essential fatty acids, for example, can retard thyroid function and brown fat activity, respectively, and compromise the body's ability to maintain its internal temperature when exposed to cold. Iodine absorption and essential fatty acid tests can reveal your status in these areas.

- **BIOMARKER 12:** *Resting Heart Rate*

This is your heart rate at rest. The best time to determine your resting heart rate is in the morning, before you get out of bed after a good night's sleep. Each of us must maintain a minimum level of cardiac output (even while at rest) in order to ensure adequate oxygenation, nourishment and waste removal for the body's cells and tissues. Your cardiac output is maintained by either a higher heart rate (if you are unfit) or by a greater "stroke volume" (if you are fit)—that is, a stronger, more efficient heart. If you are unfit, your heart must work harder by beating faster to ensure that you obtain the oxygen and nutrients that your cells, tissues and organs require. As you become more fit by following this Biological Rejuvenation Program, your heart stroke will become more powerful, thereby allowing your heart rate to slow down.

The heart beats about 60 to 80 times a minute when at rest. Resting heart rate usually rises with age, and it's generally lower in physically fit people. Resting heart rate is used to determine one's training target heart rate. Athletes sometimes measure their resting heart rate as one way to find out if they are overtraining. If you are training too strenuously, or if you have been burning the candle at both ends but are otherwise fit, your resting heart rate will begin to increase—indicating adrenal burnout or the need for rest. The heart rate adapts to changes in the body's need for oxygen, such as during exercise or sleep.

Congratulations!

If you have read these biomarkers you now have a more in-depth knowledge about the aging process than is generally taught in most medical curriculums. I do not mean to diminish in any way the training that medical doctors receive, but you now know that their focus, by definition, is on the diagnosis and treatment of disease. You also know that natural health practitioners are interested in the *prevention* and *reversal* of dis-ease so their patients can enjoy the highest possible level of health. The coolest thing is the information you've learned from the Fit Fun & Fabulous Program can help you prevent disease! I told you information is power, but remember, it is applied information that is POWERFUL!

The same holds true with accelerated aging. Through the parameters that Tuft's University has described, if we can spot areas of accelerated aging, then we can reverse that process and maintain our biological youth. Yes, we will all age, and we will all die ... this is the natural cycle of life. I often say that we live in a consumption universe—ashes to ashes—but we can also feel FIT and experience a FUN and FABULOUS life while we are on this beautiful planet. By offering this Biological Rejuvenation Program, my wish is for you to awaken every morning with the desire to live your life with joy, purpose and passion!

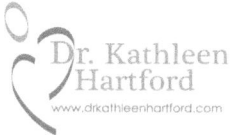

MY LIFE RE-ASSESSMENT

It is time to re-evaluate your life. Remember my experience with thousands of patients has been that when we change the physical body, we create change throughout the entire being. Did that happen for you? Please re-do this assessment on a scale of 1 to 10.

10 = Perfect bliss and happiness in relation to this area

1 = Hopelessness and impending doom in this area

Instructions

Get out some paper and sit quietly. If you meditate, please enter that meditative state. If you are not familiar with meditation then simply sit upright in a comfortable chair, close your eyes, take a few deep breaths and focus on the air moving into your body. Feel your lungs expanding with the breath you take in, then gently release the air and feel your lungs relaxing. As your lungs relax, your body and mind will relax. From this peaceful state, be aware of your feelings about your life and rank each of the following categories.

- **ETHICS** _____

  Now there is a powerful word! You cannot be your best self and live a fulfilled life if you have no moral or ethical principles. Integrity is our ability to keep these principles; it is your code of honor or the wholeness of who you are. Living in integrity is vitally important for you to feel good about yourself on the inside. Ethics make you worth knowing. It is important to examine the ethical values that you base your day-to-day existence on. Creating a value-based life provides an inner sense of integrity and wholeness that nothing else can replace.

- **FAMILY** _____

Family is possibly the most important area, and also the one most commonly taken for granted. I continuously remind parents of the importance and power they have in their children's lives. So many children are being raised by the television, the Internet or their peers. They are being programmed to be people you would not be proud to have raised, and that is the question: Does your relationship with your children "raise them up" to match with your values-based life? Or does it leave them at the mercy of commercials, entertainers, friends and movie themes that are not in accord with what you say your household stands for? Children crave guidance and they will seek it out. Make sure it's your guidance that is on their radar screen and in their hearts. Teach them gentle and powerful lessons based on your values.

Relationships with parents, children and spouses are not only important to society and to you as an individual—they are the safe space where we should be able to 'land' for comfort and security at the end of the day. Can you imagine the world if everyone took care of their own, providing safety and support for each other? Can you imagine the type of family you could create if you became deeply interested in who your children and spouse are and then shared in that?

- **FINANCES** _____

Now here is the American weakness. We have been trained to live above our means. Credit cards, credit lines, expensive toys ... they are all here for the taking. Yet I would venture to say that this area probably creates one of our greatest internal stressors. What if someone helped you to create a budget, set goals and held you to the task of getting out of debt? Social security will never allow you to live at your current level. In fact we cannot be guaranteed it will be available to us, because we have a government that also spends beyond it's means. As a responsible person, it is up to you to take care of yourself. Just as an athletic coach would never support an athlete in overindulging while in training, a personal coach would not allow you to over extend yourself financially. Rather they would help you to first get out of debt, then budget for what you truly desire and make certain that personal time and family vacations are a part of that budget.

- **HEALTH** _____

Everyone wants it, but few are willing to do what it takes to achieve and maintain it. I'm excited that by buying this book you are choosing to do just that! Let's be real, your body is the vehicle through which you will experience your life. If you were going on a cross-country trip, you wouldn't risk taking a broken-down vehicle. Yet we choose to live in broken-down bodies that might collapse at any moment. You will find it difficult to enjoy your life if you were racked with pain, unable to move, taking drugs to get through the day and living in a fog. As a coach, I am committed to you living your life FULL OUT, and you cannot do that with health challenges. Together, through the Fit Fun and Fabulous Program we will get your body in order so that you can get on with living your best life.

- **HOME** _____

Home is where the heart is. What shape is your home in? Do you enter it and say, "Ah, thank God I'm home!" or do you walk in and say, "Oh my God, what a mess"? Your house is a reflection of you. Is it messy or anal-retentively tidy? Is it lived in? Is the furniture comfortable or is it there just for show? Your house is like your skin, you should be comfortable in it.

- **CAREER** _____

Oftentimes, our work defines who we are. Have you ever asked yourself who you would be if you weren't a surgeon, a lawyer, a teacher or a homemaker? Do you know who you really are underneath the image you presently project? What would you like to do within your field? Do you want to continue to grow and learn? Or do you feel a deep despair, trapped in a career that no longer feels right for you or that no longer challenges and excites you?

- **EDUCATION** _____

    Have you always wanted to further your education? Are there certain conferences you should be attending to enhance your career? Would you like to begin to take unrelated classes in subjects you have always had an interest in? Are there particular books you should read? Knowledge is power and it can also be loads of fun. What are your educational goals?

- **RECREATION** _____

    Let's break down that word: re-create. This is where you get to recharge your batteries, pursue your passions and belly laugh. Recreation is vital to body, mind and spirit. It can be as simple as fishing, joining a gym or taking a dance class. Explore what brought you great joy as a child and do it! Chances are it will still be fun and you will feel like a new person when you're done.

- **SPIRITUAL** _____

    Do you believe in a power greater than you? If not, you probably spend a lot of time in fear. I do not care how you connect to spirit in your life, but research and experience shows that those who do are happier, healthier and live longer.

These are the important aspects that make up this incredible journey called your life. Remember that awareness is the beginning of conscious living. Awareness of the above areas has hopefully given you an opportunity to explore where you are, who you are and how you want to be in the world. Did these areas shift for you through this biological rejuvenation process? Are there areas you would like to now work on specifically to improve even further? Treat your life as a journey. There is no destination to get to, simply constant growth and improvement of who we are as a being having this human experience. God bless and go well my friend and remember:

Live your life with joy, purpose and passion!

| **Health Enhancers /** | **Health Diminishers /** |
| **Healthy Aging** | **Premature Aging** |

Balance your eating: Protein, Carbohydrates and Fats	Processed Foods and High Carbohydrate Meals
Eat Frequently (3 meals and 2 snacks)	Skipping Meals
Exercise at least 3 Times per week	Sedentary Lifestyle
Cut Down on Stimulants	Caffeine, Sugar, High Glycemic Foods
Manage Your Stress	Stress-producing Cortisol and Adrenaline
Balance Your Hormones	Hyperinsulin Diet, Stress
GMP Balanced Supplement Support	Self-prescribed vitamins which create other vitamin deficiencies

The Biological Rejuvenation Anti-Inflammatory Food Schedule

Foods to Enjoy		Foods to Avoid	
Chicken	Tapioca	Red Meats	Alcoholic Beverages
Turkey	Buckwheat and Gluten-free products	Cold Cuts	Soda, Sweetened Beverages, Citrus
Lamb	Clear, vegetable-based broth	Frankfurters, Sausage, Canned Sausage	Dried Fruit
All Legumes	Homemade Vegetarian soups	Canned Meats	Fruit Drinks, Ades
Dried Peas	All vegetables, preferably fresh, frozen or freshly juiced	Eggs	Citrus
Lentils	Unsweetened Fruit or Vegetable Juices, Water, non-citrus herbal tea	Milk	Strawberries
Cold Water Fish (Salmon, Halibut, Mackerel)	Cereals made from Rice, Corn, Buckwheat, Millet, Soy, Potato Flour, Tapioca, Arrowroot or gluten-free flour-based products	Cheese	Cereals made from Wheat, Oat, Spelt, Kamut, Rye Barley, Amaranth, Quinoa or gluten containing products
Unsweetened, Live Culture Yogurt	Unsweetened fresh, frozen or water packed canned fruits, excluding citrus and strawberries	Ice Cream	Margarine, Shortening, Unclarified butter
Rice Milk	Cold / Expeller pressed, unrefined Olive or Sunflower Oils	Cream and Non-dairy Creamers	Refined Oils
Nut Milks	Ghee, Sunflower, Sesame, Flax, Pumpkin and Squash Seeds	All gluten containing products, including gluten containing pasta	Peanuts
Soy Beverages	Salad dressings made from allowed ingredients	Canned or Creamed soups	Salad dressings and spreads
White or Sweet Potatoes	Almonds, Cashews, Pecans, Walnuts	Creamed Vegetables or Vegetables served in casseroles	
Rice		Coffee, Tea, Cocoa, Postum	

Index of Alkaline Foods

Category	Lowest Alkaline	Low Alkaline	More Alkaline	Most Alkaline
Herbs and Spices		Herbs (most)	Spices / Cinnamon	Baking Soda
Fruits	Oranges, Apricots, Bananas, Blueberries, Pineapples, Raisins, Currants, Grapes, Strawberries	Lemons, Pears, Apples, Avocado, Blackberries, Cherries, Peaches, Papayas	Grapefruit, Cantaloupe, Honeydew, Citrus, Mango, Dewberries, Loganberries	Limes, Nectarines, Persimmons, Raspberries, Watermelon, Tangerine
Vegetables, Beans, Legumes	Brussels Sprouts, Beets, Chives, Okra, Turnip Greens, Squash, Lettuces	Potatoes, Bell Peppers, Mushrooms, Cauliflower, Eggplant, Pumpkins, Collard Greens	Kohlrabi, Parsnip, Garlic, Kale, Parsley, Endive, Mustard Green, Ginger Root, Broccoli	Lentils, Yams, Onions, Daikon, Taro Root, Sea Vegetables, Burdock, Sweet Potatoes
Nuts, Seeds, Sprouts & Oils	Avocado Oil, Seeds (most), Coconut Oil, Olive Oil, Linseed Oil	Primrose Oil, Sesame Seed, Cod Liver Oil, Almonds, Sprouts	Poppy Seeds	Pumpkin Seeds
Grains & Cereals	Oats, Quinoa, Wild Rice			
Fowl				
Meat, Fish & Shellfish				
Eggs	Duck Eggs	Quail Eggs		
Dairy				
Beverages	Ginger Tea	Green or Mu tea		
Sweeteners	Suscanat	Rice Syrup	Molasses	
Vinegar		Apple Cider		

Index of Acid Foods

Category	Lowest Acid	Low Acid	More Acid	Most Acid
Herbs and Spices	Curry	Vanilla	Nutmeg	Pudding, Jams, Jellies
Fruits	Guava, Dried Fruits, Figs, Dates, Persimmon Juice	Plums, Prunes, Tomatoes	Cranberries, Pomegranate	
Vegetables, Beans, Legumes	Spinach, Fava Beans, Kidney Beans, String Beans, Chutney, Rhubarb	Tofu, Pinto Beans, White Beans, Navy Beans, Adzuki Beans, Lima Beans, Chard	Green Peas, Peanuts, Snow Peas, Legumes (other), Carrots, Chickpeas	Soybeans, Carob
Nuts, Seeds, Sprouts & Oils	Pumpkin Seed Oil, Grape Seed Oil, Sunflower Oil, Pine Nuts, Canola Oil	Almond Oil, Sesame Oil, Safflower Oil	Pistachio Seeds, Pecans	Hazelnuts, Walnuts, Brazil Nuts
Grains & Cereals	Millet, Kasha, Triticale, Amaranth, Brown Rice	Buckwheat, Wheat, Spelt, Semolina, Teff	Corn, Rye, Oat Bran	Barley
Fowl	Wild Duck	Goose, Turkey		Pheasant
Meat, Fish & Shellfish	Vension, Fish	Lamb, Mutton, Elk, Shell Fish	Pork, Veal, Mussels, Squid	Beef, Lobster
Eggs	Chicken Eggs			
Dairy	Cream, Yogurt	Cow Milk, Goat Milk, Aged Cheese, Soy Cheese	Casein, New Cheeses	Processed Cheese, Ice Cream
Beverages	Kona Coffee	Black Tea	Coffee	Beer
Sweeteners	Honey, Maple Syrup		Saccharin	Sugar, Cocoa
Vinegar	Rice Vinegar	Balsamic Vinegar		White Vinegar

Glycemic Index

Category	Low Glycemic Index	Medium Glycemic Index	High Glycemic Index
Breads, Grains, Pastas	Linguine, Multigrain Bread, Macaroni, White Spaghetti, Meat Filled Ravioli, Whole Wheat Spaghetti, Protein enriched Spaghetti, Barley, Bulgur, Chickpeas, Hominy, Parboiled Rice, Rye, Pumpernickel Bread, Rye Bread, Whole Rye, Vermicelli, Durum	Whole Meal Bread, Rye Flour Bread, Macaroni & Cheese, Hamburger Bun, Pita Bread, Brown Rice, Cornmeal, Coucous, Sweet Corn, Amylose, Gnocchi, Rice Vermicelli, Croissant	Baguette, Brown Rice Pasta, Instant Rice, Bagel, White Bread, Whole Wheat Bread, Millet, White Rice, Kaiser Roll, Dark Rye Bread
Fruits	Bananas, Kiwi, Grapes, Oranges, Peaches, Plums, Pears, Apples, Dried Apricots, Grapefruit, Cherries, Plums, Strawberries, Strawberry Jam	Pineapples, Raisins, Apricots, Mangoes, Fruit Cocktail, Canned Apricots, Apricot Jam, Cantaloupe, Mangoes, Papaya	Dried Dates, Watermelon
Snacks	Potato Chips, Chocolate, Banana Cake, Peanuts, Fruit Bread, Pound Cake, Sponge Cake	Mars Bars, Ryvita, Wheat Crackers, Popcorn, Oatmeal Cookies, Shortbread Cookies, Rye Crackers, Stoned Wheat Thins	Pretzels, Jelly Beans, Graham Crackers, Vanilla Wafers, Kavli Crackers, Saltines, Water Crackers
Cereals	Porridge, All Bran	Shredded Wheat, Oatmeal, Mini Wheats, Museli, Oatbran, Bran Chex, Cream of Wheat, Frosted Flakes, Grapenuts, Life, NutriGrain	Rice Krispies, Cornflakes, Weetabix, Puffed Wheat, Cheerios, Corn Bran, Corn Chex, Crispix, Grapenuts, Flakes, Puffed Rice, Rice Chex
Cakes, Biscuits		Croissants, Shortbread, Unsweetened Muffins, Dansh Pastries, Angel Food Cake, Bran Muffins, Blueberry Muffins	Rice Cakes, Wafer Biscuits, Doughnuts, Waffles
Potatoes, Root Crops	Sweet Potatoes, Yams	New Potatoes, Boiled Potatoes, Beets	Parsnips, Baked Potatoes, Instant Potatoes, Potato Chips, Mashed Potatoes
Vegetables	Green Peas, Carrots (cooked), Green Beans, Peppers, Spinach, Tomatoes, Artichokes, Asparagus, Broccoli, Cauliflower, Celery, Cucumber, Lettuce		
Legumes	Baked Beans, Chickpeas, Haricot Beans, Butter Beans, Lentils, Kidney Beans, Soy Beans, Baby Lima Beans, Black Beans, Brown Beans, Butter Beans, Navy Beans, Pinto Beans, Red Lentils		
Dairy	Low-Fat Milk, Fruit Yogurt, Skim Milk, Soy Milk, Low-Fat Yogurt	Low Fat Ice Cream	Ice Cream
Sugars	Lactose, Fructose	Table Sugar, Sucrose	Maltose, Glucose, Honey
Beverages	Grapefruit Juice, Pineapple Juice, Unsweetened Apple Juice, Agave Nectar	Soft Drinks, Colas, Orange Juice	Gatorade

MEAL AND SNACK SUGGESTIONS

See the Fit Fun & Fabulous Cookbook for recipes

NOTE: For "clean foods," see the Foods to Enjoy *list on the* Anti-inflammatory Food Schedule

Breakfast

- Any of our meal replacement/detoxification drinks are excellent choices for breakfast.
- Organic yogurt with granola.
- Oatmeal or any non-gluten grain. Add a scoop of rice protein powder.
- Organic egg poached, soft boiled with whole grain toast, or omelet with veggies.
  (Organic eggs are a must. The eggshell is porous so you do not want an egg that has been sprayed with toxic chemicals.)
- Fresh fruit.
- Fresh fruit smoothie.

Lunch and Dinner

- Grilled fish or chicken with vegetables.
- Salad tossed with your favorite veggies and your choice of clean protein (olive oil and lemon dressing).
- Create a stir-fry or lightly sautéed vegetables. Combine with a small portion of rice and add some high quality nuts or chicken.

- Sweet potato with tofu and asparagus. Add some pine nuts or walnuts.
- Butternut squash with cauliflower and ghee (clarified butter), sprinkle with cinnamon and pine nuts. Enjoy with broiled fish or grilled tofu.
- Greek salad with feta cheese.

Snacks
- Any and all meal replacement drinks
- Fresh fruit or fruit smoothie
- Raw vegetables dipped in hummus
- Nuts and seeds such as raw almonds, sunflower seeds, cashews, pecans, walnuts
- Ultra meal bars and protein fusion bars from our rejuvenation line

Be creative and enjoy your food. If you work in an office, consider making extra food for dinner the night before and take the leftovers to work for lunch. Keep snacks available at all times. Carry nuts or a meal replacement bar in your purse, pocket or briefcase. Have a snack every 3 hours. If you avoid hitting the "I'm starving" phase of the day it will be much easier to plan and eat the healthy suggestions above.

Consider investing in a slow cooker, which allows you to make clean stews and healthy dishes while you are at work or at the gym.

It is such a blessing to have the food availability we have in the United States, and after a few short weeks, you will be feeling the effects of clean food and a well-tuned body!

A FINAL WORD FROM THE AUTHOR

*To keep the body in good health is a duty ... otherwise we
shall not be able to keep our mind strong and clear.*
                                                    –The Buddha

*F*it, *Fun and Fabulous* is one of three books that I am creating to
support others in their personal journey. Practicing as a healthcare
provider for more than 24 years, I have seen so many people suffer due to a
lack of knowledge or understanding about how their bodies function, what
their bodies need and how to best provide for their physical health and well
being.

We are not, however, just physical beings. We also have a mental
body and a spiritual essence, all of which come together to create this
journey called "life." For this reason, I have two other books in the works.
Ramblings of a Mad Woman where we will explore the human mind and
our programmed belief systems. Rounding out the trilogy will be *What
If*, in which I will explore the exciting possibilities inherent in those two
little words. What if we are more powerful than we know? What if we are
all related? What if everyone you meet is destined to reflect back to you
an important learning? What if?

The sentiment expressed by Budda at the top of the page is very
important and very true. I do believe that until you are able to incorporate
a health supportive lifestyle (such as the *Fit, Fun and Fabulous* program),
you will be so focused on your physical ailments that you will miss the

more exciting aspects of your life. So start here, and if this is all you choose to do then that is great! You can live a life rich with energy, vitality and health. If you choose to do the entire journey with me, I would be especially happy and honored to share that experience with you.

God bless and go well –

Kathleen

ABOUT THE AUTHOR

For more than two decades, Dr. Kathleen A. Hartford has treated and nurtured thousands of individuals through her integrated wellness approaches. As patients reclaim their health, she coaches them on how to maintain their youthful vitality with practical guidance on nutrition, exercise and stress management.

She is the author of *Fit, Fun & Fabulous at Any Age* which, along with its companion journal and cookbook, creates a lifestyle approach that reverses the biomarkers of aging. This program will jumpstart anyone on their road to health and vitality. Her on line "Key to Vital Living, Healthy Aging and Weight Loss Program" has been embraced by patients across the U.S., Canada, and as far away as South Africa.

Dr. Hartford, the president and founder of Health Pyramid Longevity and Vitality Center in the Pittsburgh suburb of Natrona Heights, Pennsylvania, is also the founder of the philanthropically based *Sister Support* organization, which is dedicated to improving the lives of women through education, self-knowledge and sharing. Dr. Hartford's practice is based on balancing the five aspects of health: emotional, neurological, bio-chemical, bio-energetic and spiritual. She has been an integrated healthcare practitioner since graduating from Sherman College of Straight Chiropractic in 1986. She graduated from the University of Pittsburgh in 1978.

With an international audience, Dr. Hartford enjoys hosting the online *Key to Vital Living Radio Show & Podcasts*, and is the author of the book *Ramblings of a Mad Woman*. Dr. Hartford speaks all over the world to promote understanding among the healing disciplines and to help individuals reclaim their health in a powerful way. She has logged thousands of postgraduate hours studying Chinese Medicine, Functional Nutrition, and Neurological Repatterning, and tens of thousands of hours applying this knowledge to enhance her patients' lives. She has received numerous certifications in these techniques, including a Healthy Aging, Actual Age Certification.